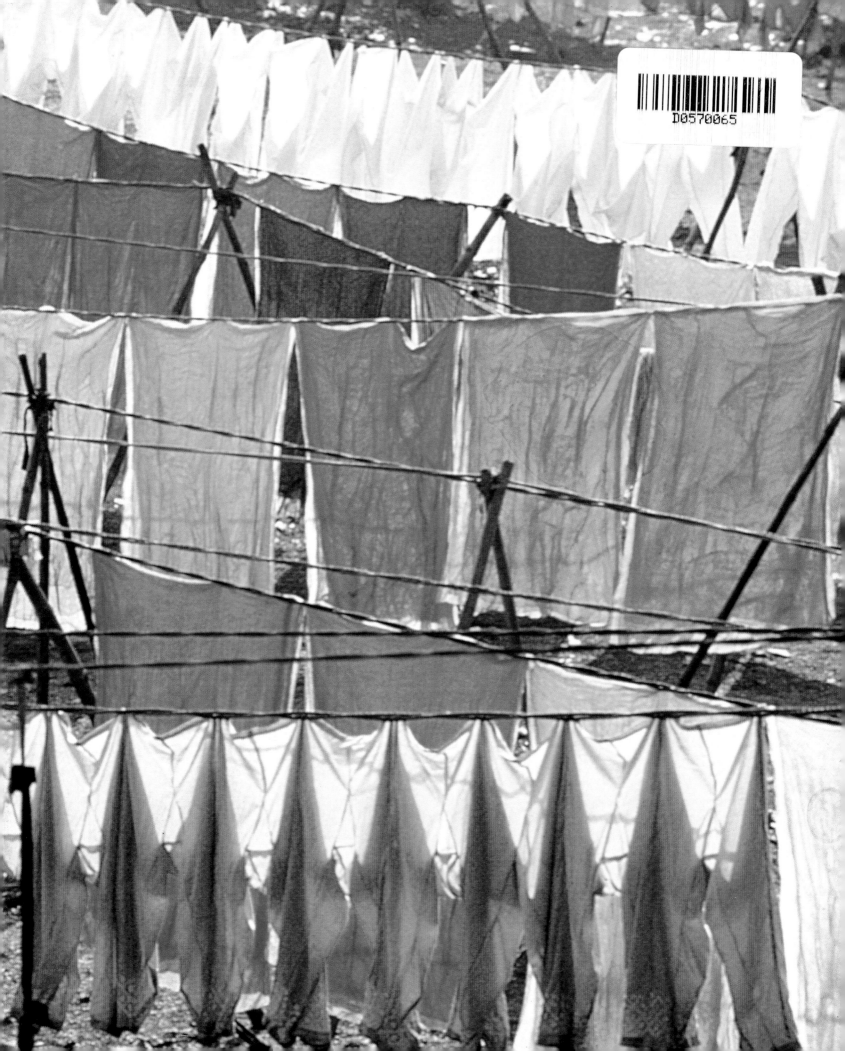

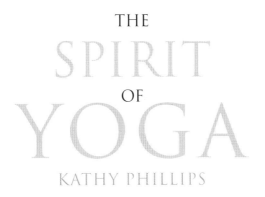

THE

SPIRIT

OF

YOGA

KATHY PHILLIPS

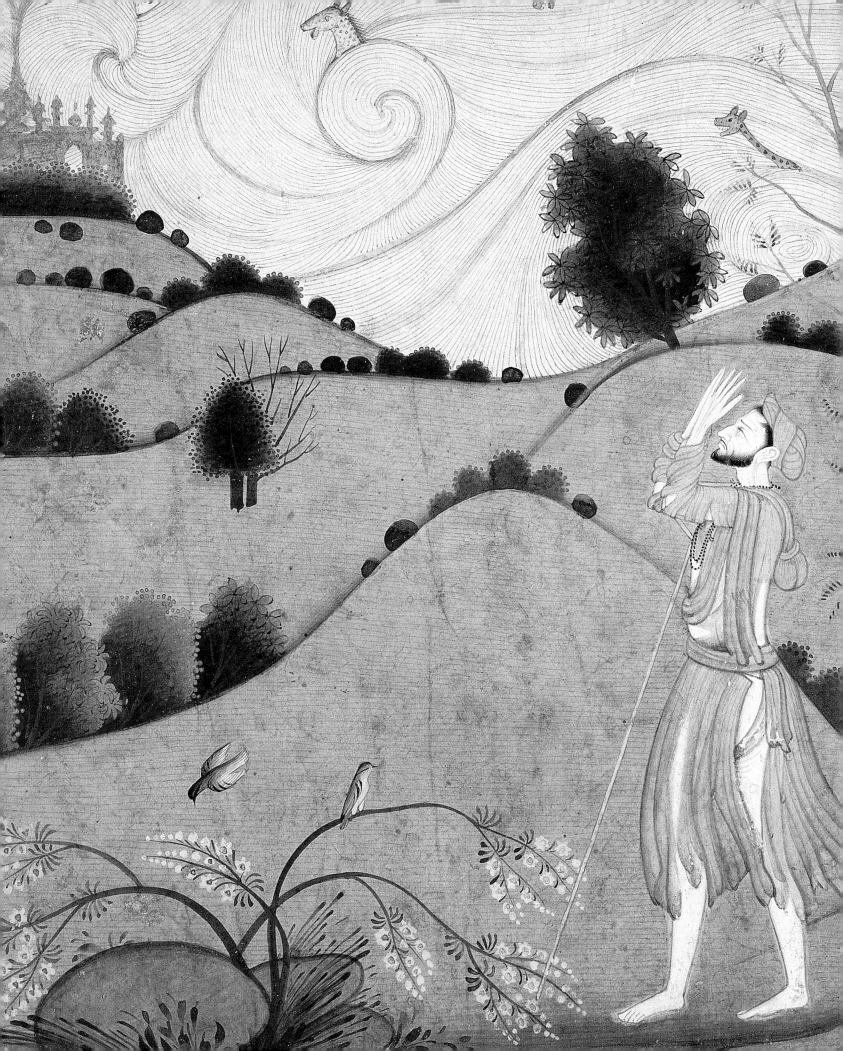

THE
SPIRIT
OF
YOGA

KATHY PHILLIPS

WITH A FOREWORD BY
CHRISTY TURLINGTON

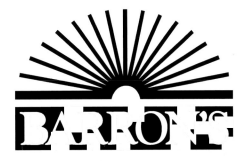

For Mary Stewart, for her wisdom, generosity and friendship.

CONTENTS

7   FOREWORD BY CHRISTY TURLINGTON

9   INTRODUCTION

11 ACKNOWLEDGMENTS

1 YOGA NOW

14 FROM HIPPIES TO THE CELEBRITY AGE

28 THE LEGACY OF THE THEOSOPHISTS

36 WHICH YOGA? DIFFERENT SCHOOLS

50 YOGA AS THERAPY

58 ECHOES OF YOGA

2 PRACTICING YOGA

64 ASANAS:

  ~ HOW ASANAS WORK

  ~ GUIDELINES FOR SAFE PRACTICE

  ~ THE ASANAS POSE BY POSE

122 PRANAYAMA:

  ~ KRIYAS, BANDHAS AND MUDRAS

  ~ THE ART OF BREATHING

  ~ SOME PRANAYAMA EXERCISES

130 MEDITATION:

  ~ DHARANA, DHYANA, SAMADHI

3 BACK TO THE ROOTS OF YOGA

138 INDIA

144 THE FIRST SONGS: THE VEDAS

150 THE FIRST POEMS: THE EPICS

158 THE FIRST INSTRUCTIONS: THE SUTRAS

170 THE EIGHTFOLD PATH

178 YOGA GROWS UP: THE SCHOLARS

184 INTIMATIONS OF IMMORTALITY

188 GLOSSARY OF SANSKRIT TERMS

189 FURTHER READING

190 INDEX

192 CREDITS

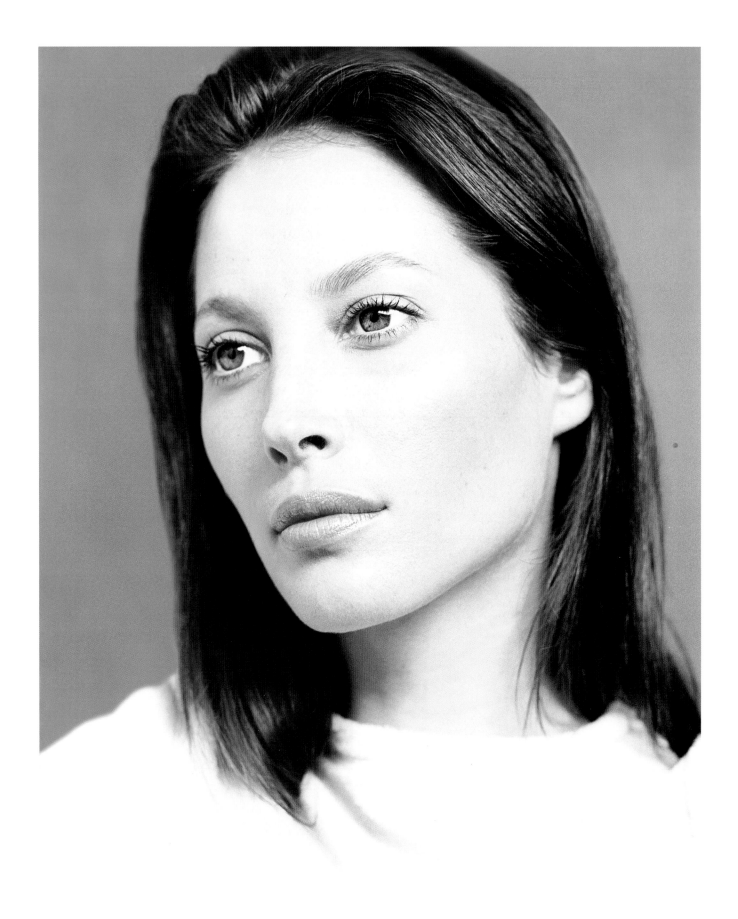

IN THE OFTEN too accurately portrayed industry of beauty and fashion, there are all sorts of contradictions. I am always asked with amazement, "Were you drawn to yoga because of the vacuous world you were in?" The answer is simple: "Yes and no." I was fourteen when I began my career as a model, and eighteen when I discovered yoga. My life had begun to be extremely frenetic and as the momentum picked up, the further behind I seemed to be leaving my body and soul. I can't say for certain whether it was what I was doing for a living as much as how and at what speed I was doing it that created this feeling of separation from myself, which in turn stirred the desire for self-realization that yoga offers. I wouldn't have had one without the other, that's for sure. Inside this world, as in many others, there are numerous paths from which to choose. My career path was loaded with obstacles, but, without them, I may never have found yoga, and, without yoga, I would not be who I am.

One of the most important things that yoga can teach us is how to discriminate and how to find equanimity in all things. It can often feel as if doing the right thing is the more difficult path to take, but the resistance itself is often the most important lesson for us – a chance to stand back and look at a situation objectively before acting. Every opportunity offers us a choice and every choice a teacher. Yoga is also something that requires practice. With the practice come many rewards. Perceptions of limitation dissolve and possibilities become endless. The industry of beauty and fashion has provided me with countless chances to exercise what yoga has taught me and has also introduced me to a few exemplary veterans, such as Kathy Phillips. Her approach to beauty has come through her longtime commitment to yoga and the light it has ignited within her, which continues to touch many others in turn through her work at *Vogue*.

CHRISTY TURLINGTON, 2001

FOREWORD

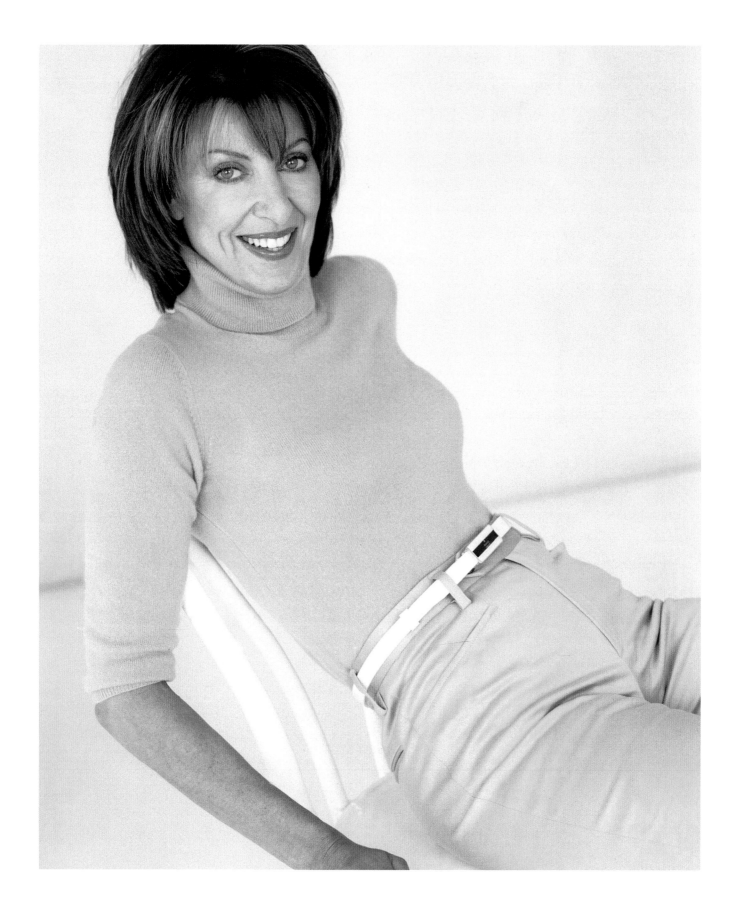

THE FIRST YOGA BOOK I EVER BOUGHT, as have thousands of aspiring yogis, was B.K.S. Iyengar's *Light on Yoga*. It was in paperback – I say was, it still is; it's just that after more than twenty-five years of use (it has traveled with me all over the world) it is in many pieces and held together with an elastic band. The other book I travel with is *Teach Yourself Yoga* by my own teacher, Mary Stewart, who has somehow managed to squeeze into this slim volume all you need to know to get to grips with the essentials of the subject, and has given invaluable advice on poses, how to do them, and why. Meanwhile the shelves of bookstores groan under the proliferation of yoga books. So what more could I have to say?

This book does not attempt to be yet another manual, another "How To" book on the vast subject of the various techniques of yoga. There are no venerable Indians in loincloths distorting themselves into inconceivable positions, nor are there athletic women in pink leotards showing the way. I wanted to make a book that was first and foremost inspirational, one that would encourage those who are interested in yoga to take it up, and at the same time enrich the practice of those who have been doing it for years.

I also wanted to decipher the mixed messages that are all over the media and in the innumerable yoga studios of every Western city in this era of global enthusiasm for the ancient Eastern art. What yoga are you studying? Just what is the difference between Hatha and Iyengar, Sivananda or Ashtanga? Can its doctrine translate with any authenticity to life in the West? Iyengar, still teaching in his eighties, said recently, "It pains me to see this great subject being commercialized and practiced superficially for show. As the winds of yoga are blowing strongly, some yoga teachers advertise their way of teaching as authentic and unique, and yet there is no depth in their sadhana."

I feel that lost in much of today's popular, acrobatic power style is the natural and lyrical flow that the body finds in the poses when they are done with humility, instinct, and using gravity. I wanted people to see a real cobra when they rise up into Cobra pose, and feel all the rootedness of a tree as they move into Tree pose. There is a history behind these poses, not only a remedial one where the organs and nervous system are massaged but an organic one from the plants, animals, and mythical heroes that inspired them. As I read up on the poses and began to write, I found that my own practice was benefiting from this approach.

INTRODUCTION

Last, but not least, I wanted to illustrate the visual and historical elements of the country and the culture that gave birth to yoga. But it was essential to me that, even when I was attempting to explain the complexities and depths of Indian philosophy, the text should remain straightforward and clear, demystifying the subject, as far as possible, to make it accessible. And if I could have had a book that you could smell, taste, and hear as well as see, I would have soaked these last pages particularly in spices, incense, and the sounds of India to give the atmosphere that I feel is part of the ancient system.

Over the past twenty-five years I have attended yoga classes all over the world. I've done yoga in moldy basements, in Zen gymnasiums, in chilly church halls, in cramped hotel rooms, and by the side of a Tiffany-blue sea. I have woken at dawn and driven from London to Oxford for regular classes, been on yoga weekends in the country, and tried classes in India, Thailand, New York, Los Angeles, Paris, and London. I have done days of yoga, three- and five-hour sessions, and forty-minute bursts; classes before and after work and in my spare time; classes where incense sticks were burned, where there was yogic jumping, Sanskrit chanting, mystic breathing and meditation; classes calling themselves Kundalini, Iyengar, Sivananda, and Hatha fusion; classes on my own and classes attended by up to a hundred people. I took up yoga having trained in ballet and turned to aerobics and jazz dance. Bored with repetitious exercise, I found that yoga worked my body safely, thoroughly, and thoughtfully, but also taught a philosophy of calm, mindfulness, and moderation. It was something of a revelation.

There is a traditional belief in yoga that you will find the right teacher for you when you need one. In that case I am blessed. My first teacher, Penny Nield-Smith, was one of Iyengar's first European pupils, whom he trained to teach in the United Kingdom. One day she sent me away from the class telling me she had taught me all she could. Almost immediately I found Kofi Busia, a Nigerian teaching in Oxford, England, whose style of yoga was tough but inspiring. I almost cried at the beginning when other people in his class stayed in Headstand for twenty minutes without any struggle. But with practice, of course, I mastered a patience and endurance that surprised me – and my friends and family. On many weekends I was up before six and driving to Oxford for his classes. I ate only macrobiotic food and forced my long-suffering family to eat molasses instead of sugar and agar agar rather than gelatin, imposing on them all manner of stringent nutritional disciplines. When Kofi moved to America, I seemed effortlessly to fall into Cathie Janson's gentle and flexible hands. With Cathie, I learned to slow down, to be more moderate, to accept. It was she who sent me to Mary when I wanted more instruction, and Mary who encouraged me to take her two-year teacher-training course. Only the other morning, while writing this book and before going to the office, I got up and did about forty minutes of practice. After my warm-up I did a Headstand, and from Headstand went into Lotus in Headstand with such ease that I amazed myself. I had thought that maybe I'd gotten to a point where my body would not progress further. And yet something had changed, given, released. There I was, all on my own with no one to share it with; and I felt gloriously happy.

The hours and years I have spent doing yoga have been a pleasure and a luxury. Time out to undo, to quiet my mind. I cannot imagine my life without it. In the end, this book is simply an attempt to share my inspirations.

KATHY PHILLIPS, LONDON, SPRING 2001

I would like to thank my editor, Rebecca Porteous, whose knowledge and enthusiasm for yoga, both in philosophy and practice, has made this book so much easier to put together. I could not have done it without her. Thanks as well to my publisher Annabel Merullo for championing me; to Mary Stewart, Chloë Fremantle, and Catherine James for constant encouragement and wisdom; and to Teresa Mermagen, who shows just how the asanas can combine strength, fluidity, and calm while looking so beautiful. Huge thanks also to photographers John Swannell, Werner Forman, Robin Derrick, and Paul Smith for their vision and generosity; to Alexandra Shulman, Vikki Berg, and Jordana Reuben at Vogue for constant support in my day job; to Pam Mason, Fleur Clackson, my agent Araminta Whitley, Sunetra Atkinson, and Catherine Green for cheering me on; to John Frieda for sending me inspiring books; to Lisa McRory, Norma Newman, Luke Hersheshon, and Germaine for their talented contribution to the photographic shoots; to Krizia, Liza Bruce, Ronit Zilka, and Pineapple for the clothes; to Kate Stephens for her sensitive layouts; to Jenny at The Yoga Place, Barbara Heller at the Werner Forman Archive, Jo Wallace at the V&A, and photographer Robert Mort for invaluable help compiling the images and ideas; to Christy Turlington for generously writing the foreword; to Giles Eyre and Charles Greig for sharing their knowledge and love of India with me all my life; and lastly to my Zen family Anthony and Oscar, for their unlimited tolerance of my preoccupation with yoga all these years and their unconditional love.

YOGA NOW

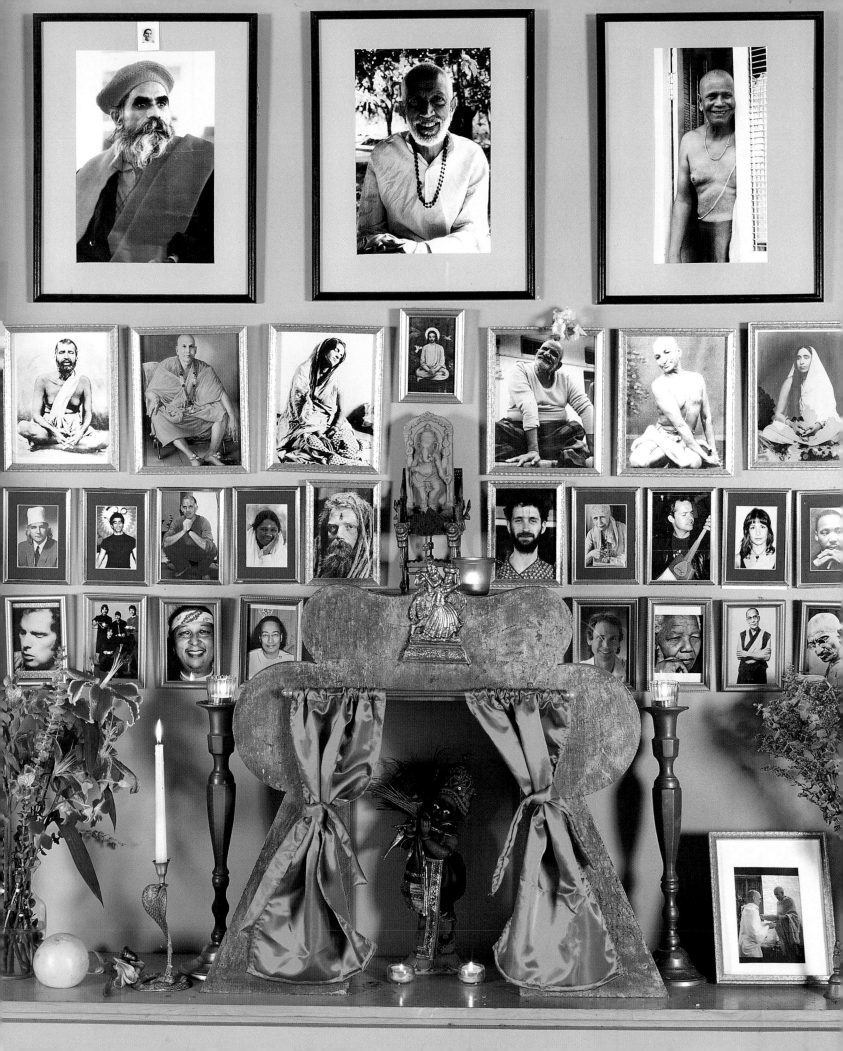

YOGA WAS DESCRIBED by the psychoanalyst Carl Jung as a form of psychic and physiological hygiene snapped up by a scattered and undisciplined public in the West mainly because of a disenchantment with formal religion and fascination for all things new. These were his reflections more than twenty years ago. What would he have had said today? How would he evaluate the super-swamis that fill yoga classes on both sides of the Atlantic, the bionic breed of contemporary yogis who boast a toned body and a working knowledge of the Hindu scriptures, their teachers who seem to have gained guru status after only a couple of years of teaching, and the now global pursuit of meditation as a panacea for all the ills and stresses of the modern lifestyle?

Even the yoga beginner has a lexicon of Sanskrit with which to impress his or her friends. In yoga classes in the United States, ritual chanting before and after class is the norm, as are the aroma of incense and the prospect of weekends on "intensives," where hours of chanting and meditation are part of the program. Classrooms, gyms, studios, and church halls are now packed with devotees, from Los Angeles to New York and from London to Sydney. Our favorite movie stars, models, designers, and TV personalities have found yoga. We read about it endlessly in the media and can snap up celebrity yoga videos, usually put together as a commercial venture with the help of a teacher who has a respectable grounding in the subject. Fashionable offices provide in-house yoga classes for the whole staff in the same way that Chinese companies offer daily T'ai Chi sessions for their employees.

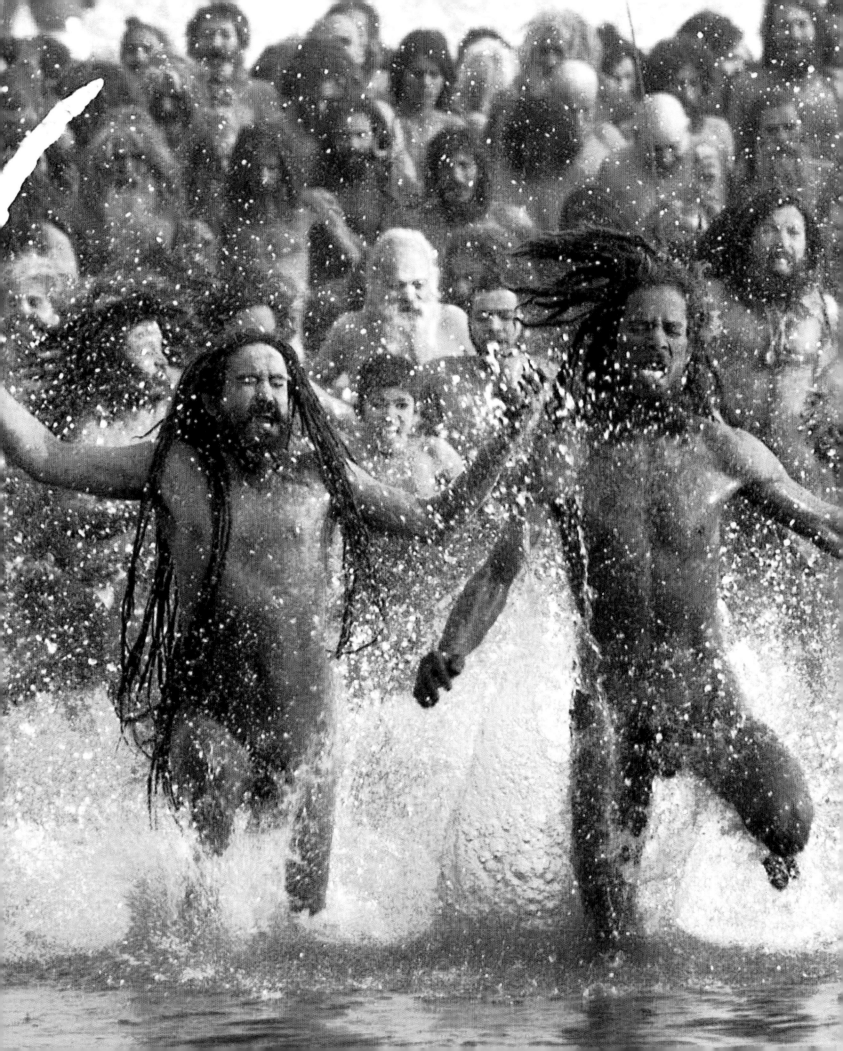

There are yoga holidays in Ibiza, Goa, and Sinai, pilgrimages to a variety of Indian ashrams, retreats to the Himalayas, and package holidays to the Indian celebration the Mela, where souls are cleansed for life by a dip in the Ganges.

The teaching of yoga is now a career prospect rather than a vocation. The members of the new yoga elite take their teachers with them wherever they go, showing off bodies that ripple with firmer muscles than any venerable Indian sage ever developed and a new philosophy of caring, sharing, and empowering. Along with this yoga lifestyle, in which an expensive organic diet is a must – but there is no restriction on alcohol and other stimulants, legal or otherwise – there are the props and costumes for the occasion, including designer yoga mats, belts, and yoga clothing with logos to authenticate them. Yes, in twenty-first-century yoga there's money to be made, not only by the gurus with their classes and intensives and membership courses, but by the selling of merchandise, tapes, how-to and philosophy books, coffee-table books (!), mugs, and t-shirts, as well as all manner of India paraphernalia, decorative trinkets and images of the gods, and so on. Just flick through one of the plethora of yoga magazines that has sprung up on newstands all over the place to see how a whole market of yoga-related consumer goods has been invented from which clever entrepreneurs are reaping profits. Hollywood has even made a movie starring none other than Madonna herself as a yoga teacher.

But how did the current explosion of interest in yoga happen? Did it spring from a renewed appreciation of all things Asian in the nineties, or had the standard career-orientated achiever simply become bored with the treadmill and weight-lifting routines in the gym or spa, and begun to explore a new way to keep the endorphin levels high?

Previous page. At this shrine at the Jiva Mukti yoga center in Manhattan, the great yogi Krishnamacharya shares a slot with The Beatles and Nelson Mandela. All are important figures in their own right, but is the juxtaposition an example of today's "supermarket" attitude to yoga and spirituality?

Left. Hundreds of Hindu holy men run into the sacred River Ganges hoping to wash away their sins on the first day of the Kumbh Mela festival, which occurs once every three years.

A man who is being delivered from the danger of a fierce lion does not object, whether this service is performed by an unknown or an illustrious individual. Why, therefore, do people seek knowledge from celebrities?

AL-GHAZALI, TWELFTH-CENTURY NORTH AFRICAN PHILOSOPHER

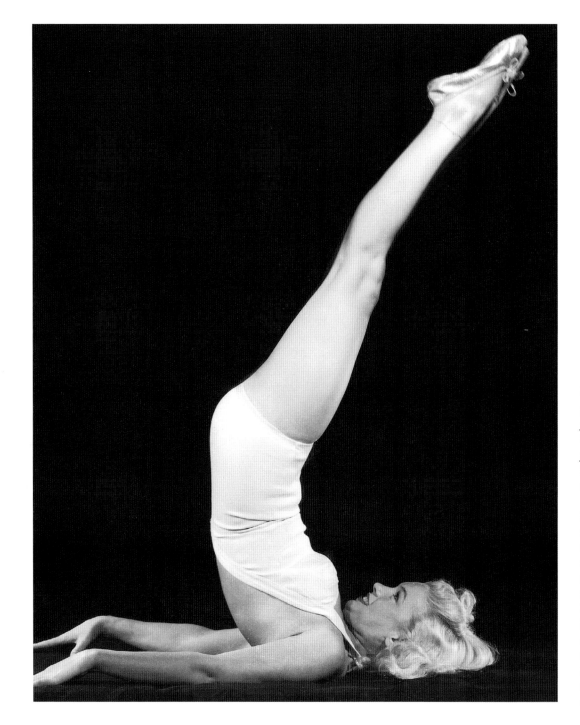

Left. Marilyn did a whole photoshoot posing in yogic postures in 1948. But no matter how much you love the Marilyn look, don't be tempted to emulate her technique.

Right. Whichever side of the Atlantic you're on, the yoga mat is the new must-have accessory, the Hermés bag of spirituality. Meg Ryan, Dennis Quaid, Gwyneth Paltrow, Julia Carling, and Madonna are some of the celebrities who have helped to turn yoga into the hottest trend in bodywork.

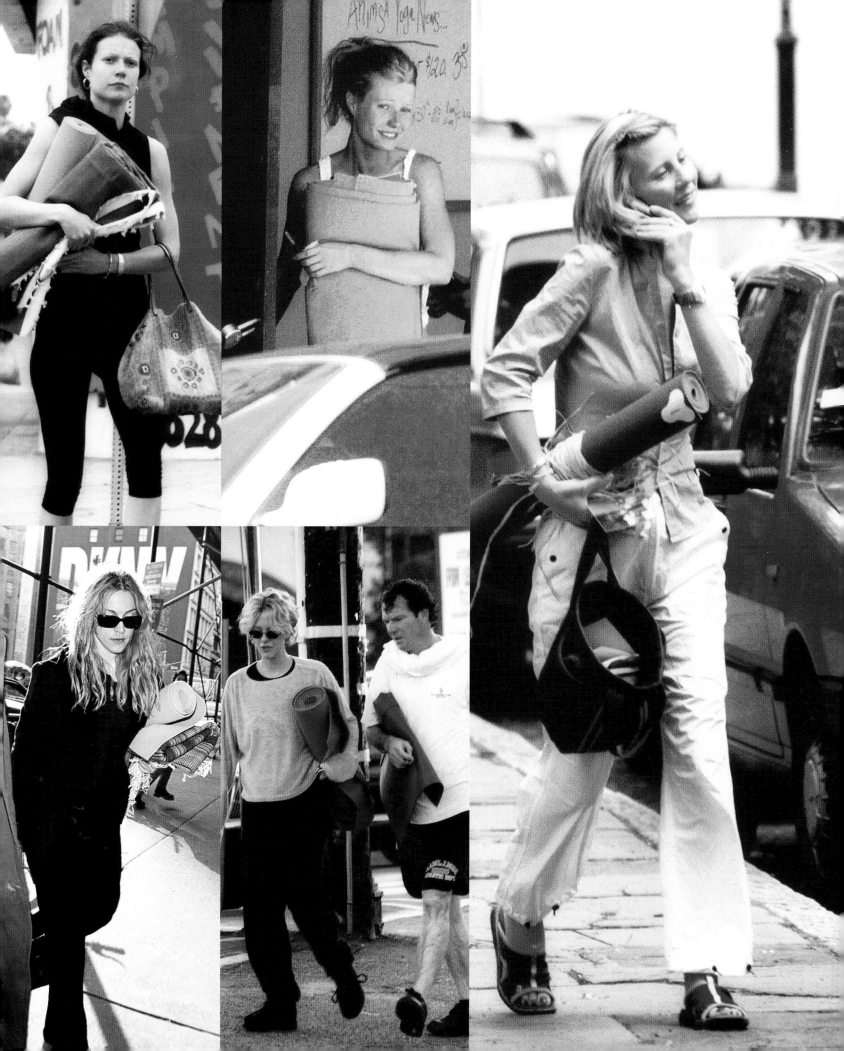

The first waves of enthusiasm for yoga were considered by the established Church to smack of evil rituals, its practitioners weird hippies and eccentrics who were anarchic, anti-establishment, and probably out of it on drugs. Today's yoga devotees are mostly respectable, middle class, bourgeois, and looking for deeper meaning in their lives. And twenty-first-century yogis are indeed evangelical about the life-changing effects of their daily discipline, just as The Beatles found themselves transformed by their meeting with Maharishi Mahesh Yogi, who, forty years ago, taught them to practice Transcendental Meditation. He opened their eyes to new ways of perception in the same way that Jiddu Krishnamurti had captivated audiences in post-war America, but neither guru thought a rigorous routine of "down dogs" and "chatarangas" a necessity. A new generation of yoga faithful, turned on by the feel-good, look-good factor that regular asana practice produces, has supplanted both the sixties' New Agers and the intellectuals in search of the truth and become fascinated by yogic philosophy along the way.

Madonna's new passion leads to a leading role. She reinvents herself as a yoga teacher in The Next Best Thing. *Here she is with co-star Rupert Everett.*

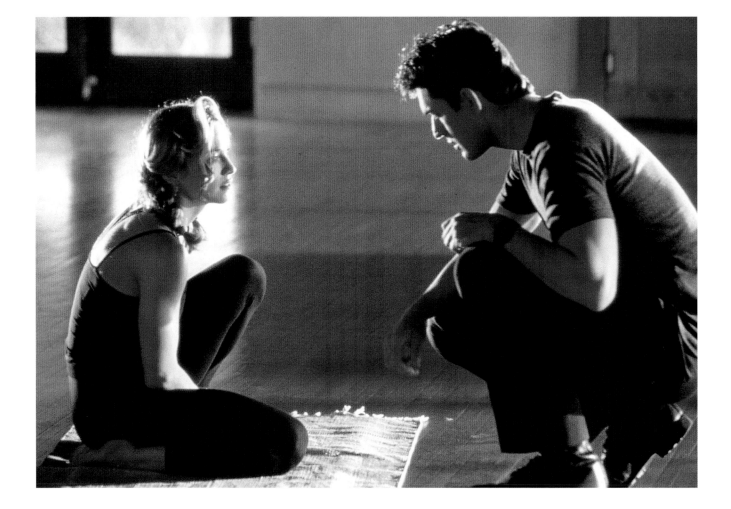

And why wouldn't they be? The Church and its influence has declined more than ever; people feel powerless in the face of globalization, pollution, ecological destruction, and market forces that sweep away all possibility of being masters of their own destinies. Even scientists, traditionally atheists to a man and once so sure of the facts, are now debating the origins of life itself. Some are saying that there may well be a God or at least some other dynamic force that is out there. They are busy rethinking the theory of relativity as well as changing their attitude to the law of gravity. If this weren't enough to unbalance us all, new research suggests that the universe is not four-dimensional, but that it might be made up of twenty or thirty dimensions. The Big Bang, physicists pronounce, might have been not the dawn of evolution but merely the start of a new era. No wonder the ancient yogic concept of "prana," which signifies both the breath and the universal dynamic of the cosmos, is an attractive image. It is, after all, a hypothesis that's been around, and not successfully challenged, for some five thousand years.

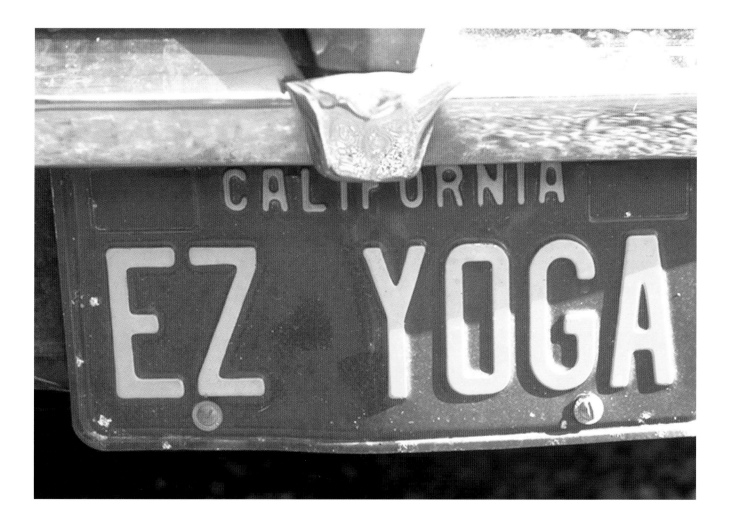

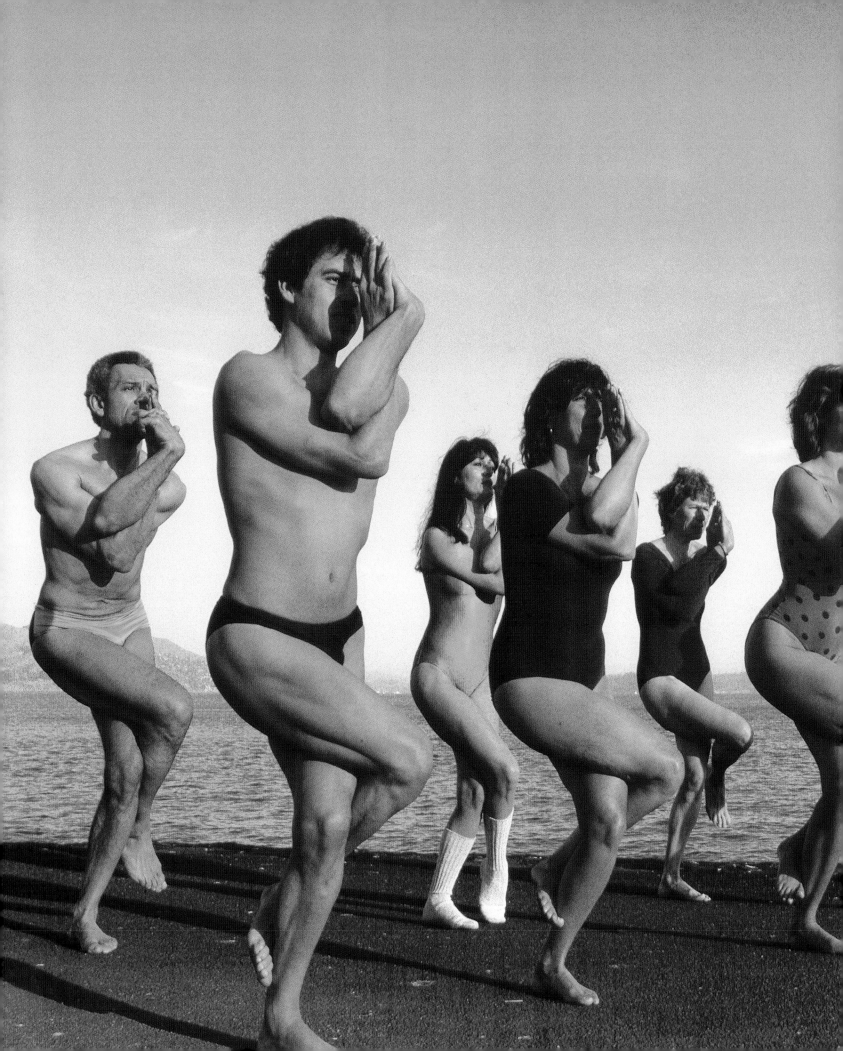

The beach has always
been a favorite spot
for group yoga, from
Bombay to Brighton,
to the beaches of
California. Yoga was
clearly a new-enough
phenomenon on British
beaches in 1934 for
these children doing
Cobra, below, to have
attracted quite a crowd.
By the 1980s it had
become such a common
sight in California that
this group of adults, left,
contorting themselves
into Eagle pose, seem
to have attracted little
more than the interest of
a passing photographer
with a sense of humor.

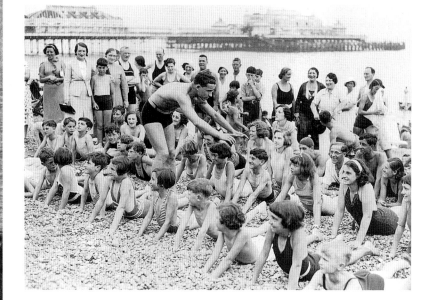

But over time, with the mingling of rituals and philosophies from a plethora of Eastern cultures, practices have changed. The new yoga, with its decidedly aggressive style, is at odds with the gentle, noncompetitive spirit of latter-day converts in the sixties and seventies. Now there is rivalry, not only between the various style factions – the type of yoga you choose to do – but also in the classroom itself. Classes are not so much places where the teacher might instruct on the subtleties of a position as they are platforms that offer a chance to perform, to impress others with a fabulous ability to balance and bend and contort the body into ever more demanding positions. Now it is about being the best you can, about being more centered, more equipped for performance. There is less emphasis on inquiry and the slow acquisition of wisdom and more on solutions to despondency and the continuation of the obsession with a beautiful body – the significant by-product of yoga. The power gym workout that originated in L.A. has segued into the power yoga workout for a new millennium and there is no question that for some this is little more than a fitness regime that has generated a trend for a new sinewy, muscled physique.

And if today's trend for so-called power yoga did come in on the back of the Californian obsession with aerobic fitness, that quest for some kind of bodily perfection as an antidote to polluting addictions, there may be a twist in the tale. When Krishnamacharya, one of the great gurus of modern yoga, was teaching the Maharajah of Mysore in the 1930s, the Maharajah, clearly a well-traveled nobleman, apparently professed an interest in Western gymnastics. It is, of course, possible that a Western gymnastic element crept into the Indian

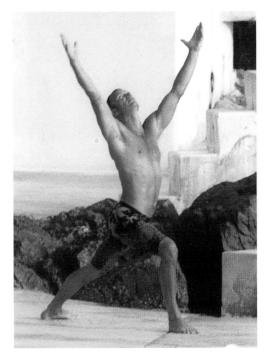

The phenomenon of so much contemporary "spirituality" is not of a pilgrimage to the center. It is more like a raid mission that descends suddenly, plunders what can be got in the form of spiritual experience or insight, and then immediately retreats behind the walls of the religious ego.
DOM JOHN MAIN

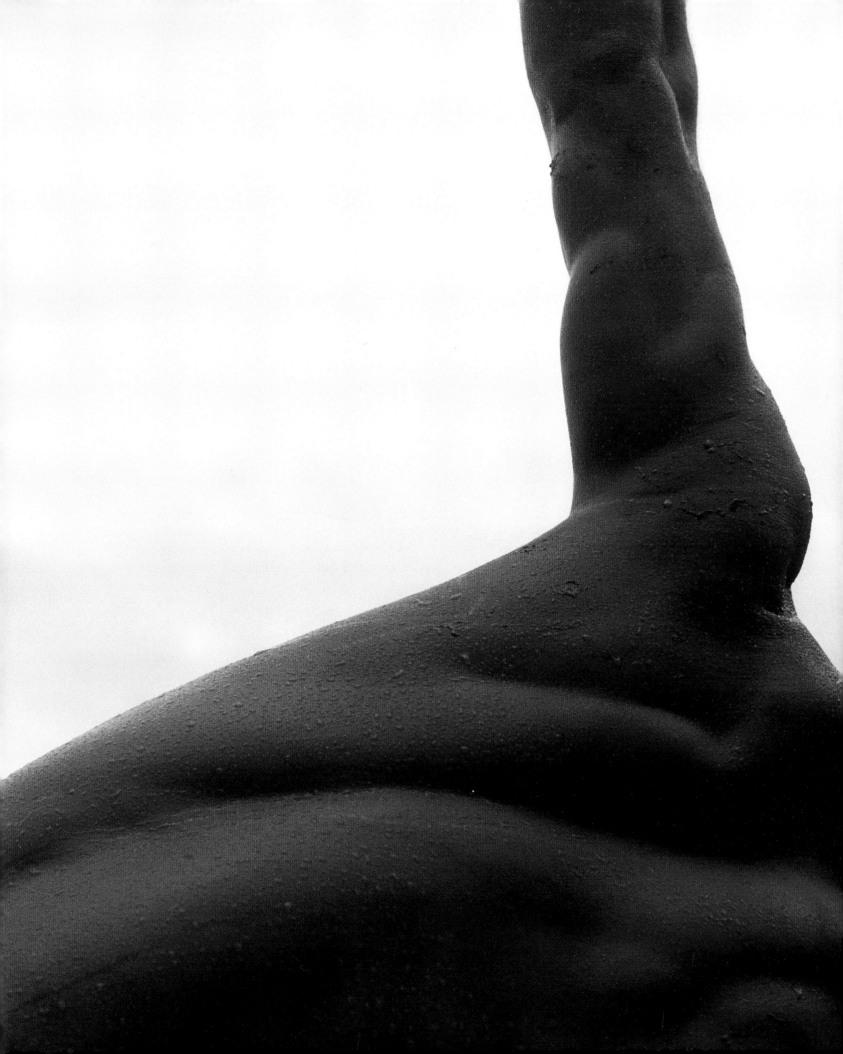

routine in the same way that little bits of T'ai chi, Feldenkrais, and aerobics have crept into current asana practice. But whatever the truth of the matter, when Krishnamacharya's disciples, particularly Pattabhi Jois, went off to America to spread the word, their instruction may not have been so authentically Eastern after all, merely their own calisthenics recycled.

Like every other Western craze, a whole set of consumer must-haves have been invented to go with yoga practice. Where B.K.S. Iyengar once claimed in his great book, *Light on Yoga*, that you needed no more than a mat and some space in the shade to be able to practice, students – and particularly Iyengar followers – now use all manner of hardware; straps, foam blocks, blankets, chairs, and specially crafted backrests push the Western body, not necessarily genetically programmed to be flexible in the same ways as its Eastern counterpart, further and further. British Indians, for many of whom yoga is part of the culture of their roots, are generally bewildered, and in some cases offended, at the way their sacred chants, costumes, and rituals have been ambushed and taken up in the United Kingdom. And, of course, just as there is a world of difference between the local Indian ashram and some of the cultist gatherings developed to cater for eager Western yoga devotees, there are Indians who are shamelessly developing programs to entice naïve enthusiasts to part with their dollars. "Who knows how much of what happens today is in the ancient spirit of yoga," muses Mary Stewart, who studied with Iyengar, has taught in England, America, Canada, Italy, and India for more than thirty years, and developed, with her friend Vanda Scaravelli, a new approach to yoga that puts more emphasis on breathing. "There seems to be a supermarket attitude to spirituality today," she says. "You can indulge yourself if you've got the time, and you can pick and mix and make up the rules as you go along."

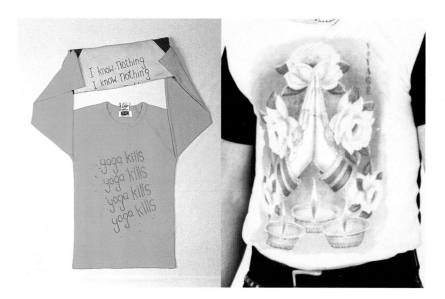

As a product to be marketed, yoga has lost its brown rice and open-toed sandal image for a touch of classic British irony or even pure kitsch.

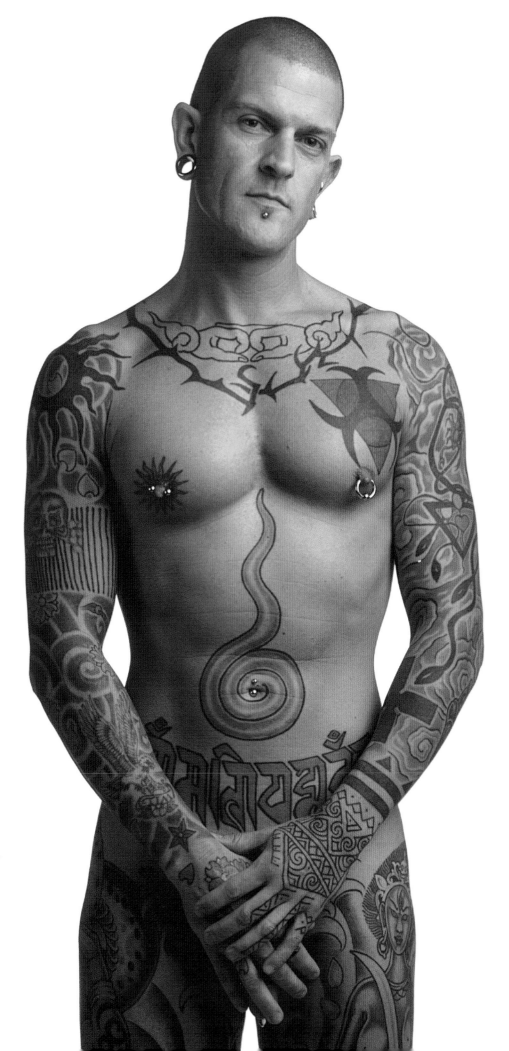

This man's body is tattooed with sacred symbols from a whole collection of Eastern mystical traditions, not least of which is the wonderful kundalini serpent coiled around his belly button and beginning its ascent to his crown chakra.

Confine the body and you shrink the Spirit. The all-new Avalon. The most spacious, luxurious sedan we've ever created. Toyota. Be good to yourself. Every Day.

TOYOTA ADVERTISEMENT, *NEW YORKER*, 1999

SOME OF THE PEOPLE who consider themselves part of this new wave of yoga may look back at the late twentieth century and see it as a time when the West developed a conscience, when a disenchantment with materialism gave way to the search for a more spiritual life. Certainly the language of such a conscience has integrated itself deep into our society over the course of the last decades of the twentieth century, as the wording for the Toyota advertisement illustrates. But even for those of us who do believe in the integrity of this contemporary New Age, it is not as new as we may think. Much of the credit for the introduction to the West of Indian religious and philosophical ideas must be given to the Theosophical Society, founded in the United States by Madame Helena Blavatsky, an eccentric woman with a mysterious background, who claimed to have aristocratic Russian origins. By the same token, most of the literary material on which the study of Indian philosophy in the West has been based was, until very recently, translated by the Theosophical Society and inevitably influenced by the Society's beliefs. The Theosophists' indirect influence on our Western understanding of Eastern philosophy has, therefore, been far greater than most people would credit.

THE LEGACY OF THE THEOSOPHISTS

IN THE EARLY 1870S Madame Blavatsky appeared in America to advance the theory that man descended from spirit beings rather than apes. Blavatsky was no "looker"; a large woman with bulging eyes, she was a forceful personality with a unique and provocative vision plus the charisma and chutzpah to influence a sizeable audience. Theosophy, which solidified into the movement she founded in 1875 with Henry Olcott, spawned innumerable rival gurus and sects, including the German philosopher Rudolf Steiner, the charismatic G. Gurdjieff, P. Ouspensky, and J. Krishnamurti. And their ideas were taken up not just by a bunch of crackpot losers but by some of the most prominent intellectuals of their time, among them Aldous Huxley, Frank Lloyd Wright, W. B. Yeats, and Christopher Isherwood, the last of whom later interpreted the Yoga Sutras of Patanjali. On the whole, however, these various societies and foundations were kept alive by the donations of the bored rich and a cast of lost souls looking for a cause to which they could belong.

In 1896 the society identified three main goals: the formation of a universal human brotherhood without distinction of race, creed, sex, caste or color; the encouragement of studies in comparative religion, philosophy, and science; and the investigation of unexplained laws of nature and the powers latent in man. The Theosophists and their students studied yogic thought and developed it either as academic science or as something almost approaching an organized religion. Their message was one of spiritual, not physical, liberation. They expounded a body of religious dogma as well as teaching certain so-called spiritual techniques designed to promote enlightenment. These included study, prayer, and meditation with the premise that only the selfless, the pure of heart, mind, and body, would be able to communicate with the spirits, or "Masters."

Thou are Thyself, the object of thy search.
BLAVATSKY

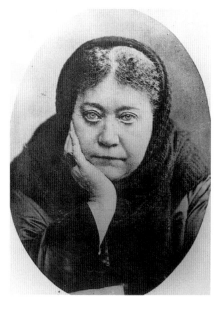

Madame Blavatsky, founder of the Theosophical Society.

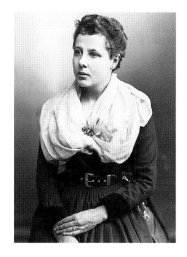

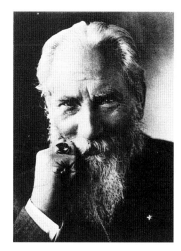

Annie Besant at the age of eighteen. She became head of the Theosophical Society and Krishnamurti's adoptive mother, taking over his education and upbringing.

Rudolf Steiner, the celebrated German philosopher, a one-time member of the Theosophical Society and founder of the Anthroposophical Society.

Charles Leadbeater, friend and associate of Madame Blavatsky, was eventually prosecuted in Australia, where he had taken refuge from scandals — relating to the sexual abuse of boys in his care — in Europe and India.

The mind that is seeking experience is incapable of understanding what the truth is.
J. KRISHNAMURTI

In the search for the key to the mysteries of the universe, Blavatsky claimed to have occult powers that allowed her to communicate with the Masters. Among them were all the great religious leaders of the past, including the Buddha, Confucius, Jesus Christ, Lao Tzu, and so on. Certain less well-known Masters were in communication with Blavatsky through letters, séances, and dreams, or so she maintained. The Masters lived on a higher plane, were immortal and immaterial, and could materialize whenever and wherever they liked. A central feature of Blavatsky's teaching was that an individual could develop similar occult powers to hers if he or she had the required amount of training and devotion.

Blavatsky fascinated her acquaintances with a knowledge of Asian scriptures and tales of a spiritual journey she claimed to have taken in Tibet in her youth. She took up fashionable ideas and gave them her spin, such as her belief that the excavation of Mayan and other Central American sites would prove that America had housed the oldest civilization the world had known, and that California might become the next center of world civilization and, therefore, of cosmic evolution.

These pronouncements, plus her séances, mystical correspondences in the form of pamphlets, letters, and magazines, and messages from other planes, were esoteric ideas that fascinated a late-nineteenth-century audience eager to believe in her. The jury is still out on whether or not Blavatsky was a fraud, but be that as it may, Theosophy had a radical impact on cultural, social, and even political life at the time, and was a great influence on the development of Western spiritualism through its writings, translations, and some of its one-time devotees, particularly Krishnamurti, Gurdjieff, Ouspensky, and Rudolf Steiner.

After the death of Blavatsky, the next powerful woman to run the Theosophical society was Annie Besant, who became enchanted with India – where the movement is still a force to be reckoned with – and went to live there. It was during the time that Besant lived in Banaras (then called Varanasi) that Krishnamurti was discovered, playing with his brother on a beach near Madras, by the entirely suspect and pedophiliac Charles Leadbeater. The Theosophists proclaimed him to be a second Christ and predicted that he would become a world teacher. He was taken from his family and patronized by Besant and Leadbeater, who taught him about his own culture and groomed him for his role of guru. Other second generation Theosophists, such as Ouspensky, an upper-middle-class Russian in exile, and Rudolf Steiner, the son of a stationmaster from Styria on the Austro-Hungarian border, split from Theosophy and went on to develop their own philosophies. Steiner founded the important and substantial doctrine of Anthroposophy, on which the tried and tested methods of biodynamic farming and his alternative method for teaching children are based, while Ouspensky wrote books on the themes of karma and reincarnation that still sell more than forty thousand copies a year.

The most difficult lesson to learn about caring for the soul is that our best and most cherished ambitions are its worst enemy.
THOMAS MOORE

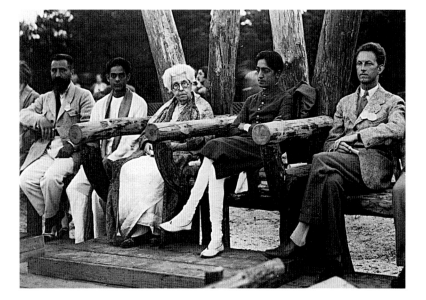

A gathering of the Order of the Star of the East. Annie Besant presides, with the young Krishnamurti sitting on her left.

Of all these figures, though, it was Krishnamurti who became the star. In between the two world wars there was a close-knit social circle of intellectuals and celebrities in the firmament around "K"'s new life in California; it included Aldous Huxley, Bertrand Russell, Christopher Isherwood, Igor Stravinsky, Iris Tree, Charlie Chaplin, and Greta Garbo. The paradox is immediately evident: a solitary guru preaching profoundly on the subjects of human frailty and of the necessity for detachment, while living cut off from his roots in that curious unreal world peopled by celebrities, pop stars, and mystical heiresses searching for the truth. Krishnamurti's status as a spiritual leader required that he lead a life of devotion and absolute chastity, which proved to be a difficult proposition for a man who grew up to be handsome, charismatic, and always surrounded by adoring females. Krishnamurti, like many other gurus before and since, failed to stay as chaste and incorruptible as was expected of a New Age Messiah. Until his death at the age of ninety-one, he declared that he deplored the guru–disciple relationship and yet he spent his time being paid to dispense a higher wisdom to a social elite willing to pay for the privilege.

Today's gurus are in much the same predicament. Take the highly intelligent Deepak Chopra, a brilliant communicator who has acquired an audience (and a fortune) by retelling the ancient Hindu and Buddhist theologies to a new celebrity following eager to change their lives, or the beautiful Gurumayi Chidvilasananda who teaches Siddha meditation. Both of them attract fervent high-profile devotees as fast as they preach truths about the pointlessness of hanging on a guru's every word.

Contemporary political philosopher Simon May has identified some qualifications for being a guru. Two of those he cites are being an outsider on

Right. Marlon Brando gets intense. Political philosopher Simon May says one qualification for being a guru is to have a capacity for contact with the ordinary "so intense that it appears to be mystical."

Far right. Deepak Chopra is a master of communication and uses the language of spirituality in a way that today's seekers can understand.

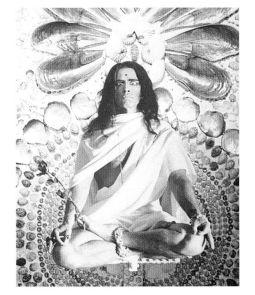

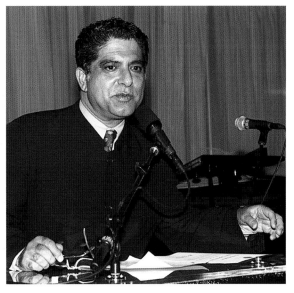

the margins of society and having a capacity for contact with the ordinary "so intense that it appears to be mystical." The guru in Indian society was above all the castes, the teacher whom kings and ministers consulted for their wisdom. Most of today's gurus appear to be associated more with opportunism, exploitation, and great wealth than anything else. In fact many of the Indian, and Tibetan, gurus who have come to the West have had their reputations tarnished by scandals both sexual and fiscal in nature. There have been stories of celibates who have strayed; of devout gurus who, when found fondling young boys, have explained that they are trying to "raise the kundalini" of their pupils; of funds having been accumulated for the acquisition of innumerable expensive cars, jewelry, and all the trappings of the material, consumer world; of priests who have admitted to molesting their charges; and of acclaimed teachers who have used their position of trust to persuade pupils that to lapse under their guidance is not a sin. In many cases, the transgressions have been overlooked, presumably on the premise that spirituality or even sanctity need not exclude sexual love, though it is impossible not to see this reasoning as hypocritical.

Alternative religions and religious teachers are as attractive today as ever. Books such as Laird T. Spalding's five volumes entitled *The Life and Teaching of the Masters of the Far East*, a work not unlike the occult pronouncements of Madame Blavatsky, are still selling all over the United States, alongside all manner of esoteric occult theories. And we must not forget the more recent publishing phenomenon of James Redfield's *Celestine Prophecy*, published in 1993 to become the number-one international bestseller for two years in a row, with global sales going well into the millions. This book of ten insights, a parable about the need for spiritual understanding in today's world, is told as a simple story involving "revelations," "synchronicity," and "materializing at will"; the message reads that living and communicating on another plane is possible through purity of thought and action. Madame Blavatsky would have been proud of it. The sales figures suggest that, more than a hundred years later, there is a still a universal hunger for the answers to the key questions of existence that neither mainstream religion nor science have satisfied. The start of a new millennium has found an even wider public hungry for spiritual adventure.

Right. A solitary figure walks the beach in India. The splendid isolation of some of India's remoter shores has long inspired spiritual seekers to look within.

People travel to wonder at the heights of mountains, at the huge waves of the sea, at the long courses of rivers, at the vast compass of the ocean, at the circular motion of the stars; and they pass by themselves without wondering.

ST. AUGUSTINE

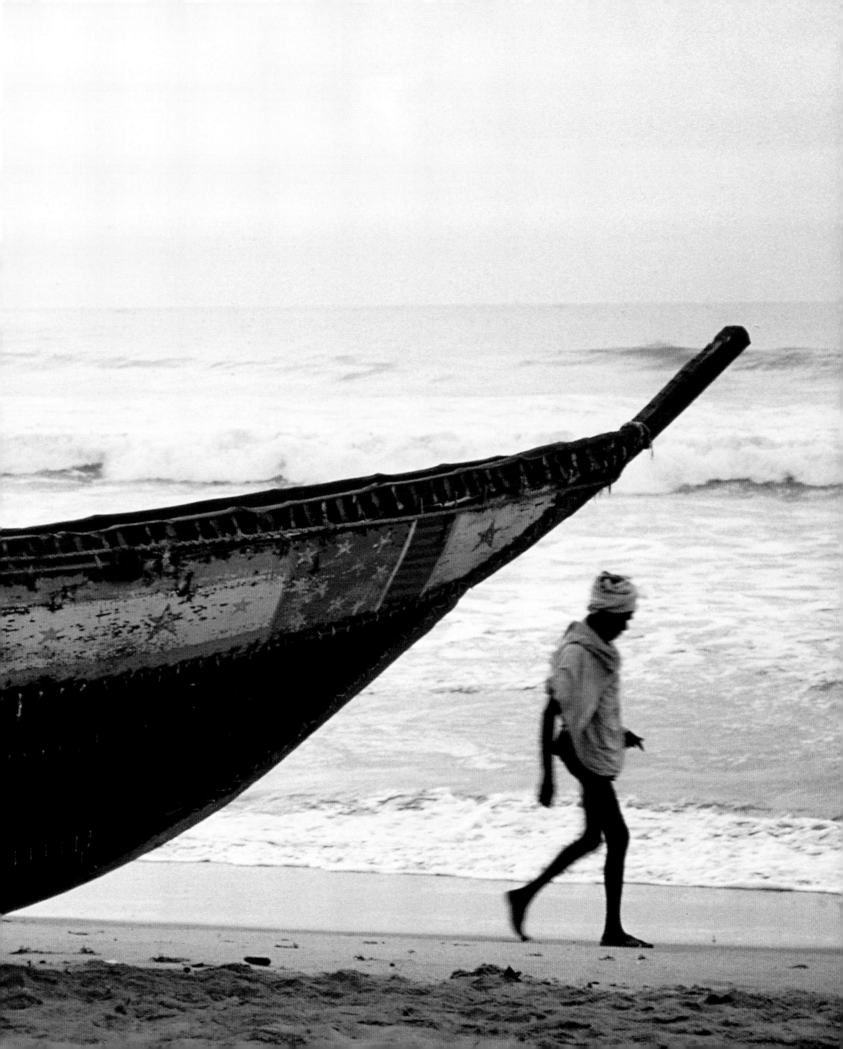

Asana practice is a concrete way to exercise equanimity of the mind.

WILLEM DAFOE, ACTOR

SCHOOLS, ashrams, and centers of yoga have proliferated all over the Western world since the start of the twentieth century. Teachers have developed techniques and changed emphasis, and then given names to their "new" methods. Like a river delta or the branches of a tree, the schools of yoga continue to ramify into still more schools. Today there are so many to choose from it can be difficult to know where to start. The term "yoga" is now applied to many forms of asceticism, meditation, and spiritual training, but originally it came from southern India as a discipline whose aim was to escape the karmic cycle of cause and effect and reach a higher consciousness. The *Bhagavad Gita* names eighteen different kinds of yoga, each with its own emphasis. The Yogatattva (Sanskrit scripture) recognizes four kinds – Hatha Yoga, Laya (or Kundalini) Yoga, Mantra Yoga, and Raja Yoga. But Jnana Yoga, Bhakti Yoga, Kriya Yoga, Tantra Yoga, and Karma Yoga are often mentioned. These "paths" should not be confused with "schools" of yoga, which are a modern phenomenon, named to distinguish the teaching style of one guru or establishment from another. Famous "brands" include Iyengar and Sivananda. To add further confusion, some schools of yoga appropriate Sanskrit words that define aspects of traditional yoga paths as their names. Ashtanga yoga, for example, gets its name from the eightfold ashtanga path set out in Patanjali's Yoga Sutras. But today more people know it as the fast, athletic power-yoga first taught by Pattabhi Jois in Mysore and New York.

KRISHNAMURTI FOUNDATION

VARIOUS VEDANTA SOCIETIES

The first of the Vedanta Societies, the Western branches of the Ramakrishna Order, was established in New York in 1894.

Swami Vivekananda
1863–1902
Disciple of Ramakrishna and, in 1893, the first person to take yoga to the World Parliament of Religions.

RAMAKRISHNA ORDER
Founded by Ramakrishna, 1836–1886.

Krishnamurti
1894–1986
One of the great iconoclasts of the last century and a powerful spiritual leader in his own right.

Swami Prabhavanda
Head of the Ramakrishna Order in Los Angeles in 1899.

ASHTANGA YOGA

The Theosophical Society is still active all over the world, principally in India.

Annie Besant
1847–1933
Head of the Theosophical Society after Madame Blavatsky died.

THEOSOPHICAL SOCIETY
Founded by Madame Blavatsky and Henry Olcott in 1875. An influential and widespread movement that had many offshoots, and was largely responsible for the exposure of Indian philosophy and philosophical literature to the Western world in the first half of the twentieth century.

Pattabhi Jois
b.1918
Founded Ashtanga Yoga Institute in Mysore in 1948.

ANTHROPHOSOPHICAL SOCIETY
Founded by the German philosopher Rudolf Steiner.

10

VINIYOGA

T.K.V. Desikachar
b.1938
Krishnamacharya's son; opened Krishnamacharya Yoga Mandiram in Madras in 1976.

Krishnamacharya
1891–1989
Remarkable for his learning and for the variety of schools of yoga that stemmed from his teaching.

Sri Ramamolan Brahmachari
Krishnamacharya's guru in Tibet.

B.K.S. Iyengar
b.1913
Krishnamacharya's brother-in-law; founded Ramamani Memorial Institute in Pune in 1973.

Indra Devi
b.1899
Krishnamacharya's first Western pupil.

Guru Ram Das
1534–1581
The fourth Sikh guru.

9

KUNDALINI YOGA

IYENGAR YOGA
Centers established worldwide.

INDRA DEVI FOUNDATION
Based in Switzerland.

Yogi Bhajan
b.1929

8

A doctrine that insists that the body is the means rather than the obstacle to enlightment. It has a huge influence on both Hinduism and Buddhism, and provides an obvious link with Hatha Yoga, where the emphasis is also on the body. _____

Mary Stewart
Diana Clifton
Silva Mehta
Vanda Scaravelli

Gurmukh Kaur Kalsa
Los Angeles–based teacher to the stars and disciple of Yogi Bhajan.

3HO Foundation
Established in California in 1969 by Yogi Bhajan.

Lihar Po
Tibetan White Tantra teacher.

7

Shankara was a scholar _____ of Vedanta and orthodox Brahminism, who articulated the non-dualist model of reality, and spawned many monastic lineages, in which several modern schools of yoga find their origins.

WHITE TANTRA

6

Tenzin Warigyal Rinpoche

TRUL-KHOR

TIBETAN YOGA
Revered yogis in the Buddhist tradition include Naropa, a renowned master of Tantric Buddhism, and Milarepa, the greatest poet, mystic, and hermit in the religious history of Tibet.

Milarepa
d.1122

Naropa
d.1040

5

FIVE RITES OF REJUVENATION

YANTRA YOGA

One of the two _____ great epics, the *Mahabharata* contains the *Bhagavad Gita*.

4

The Five Tibetans

Chogyal Namkhai Norbu
b.1938

3

Seals dug up from sites of the _____ ancient Indus Valley civilization show people in poses that are identifiable yoga asanas, such as mulabandhasana and baddha konasana.

2

1

SIDDHA YOGA

Dates back to 9th-century Kashmiri Shaivism, and is based on aphorisms told to Vasugupta by Shiva.

Bhagawan Nityananda
1896–1961

Swami Muktananda
1908–1982

Swami Chidvilasananda
b.1955

Otherwise known as Gurumayi, she heads what is now officially called the Siddha Yoga Meditation Institute.

Baba Hari Dass

Called his yoga "Ashtanga Yoga", after Patanjali's eightfold path. (Not to be confused with the newer "Ashtanga Yoga" expounded by Pattabhi Jois.)

Mount Madonna Center

Ashram in California.

KRIPALU YOGA

Inspired by Swami Pranavananji.

KRIYA YOGA

SELF-REALIZATION FELLOWSHIP

Inspired by Paramahansa Yogananda.

Swami Pranavananji

Believed to be an incarnation of Shiva.

Lahiri Mahasya
1827–1895

Swami Kripavanji
1913–1983

Sri Yukteswar
1855–1936

Amrit Desai
b.1932

Paramahansa Yogananda
1893–1952

Brother of Bishnu Ghosh and author of the world-famous *Autobiography of a Yogi.*

Swami Satchaidananda

Swami Satchaidananda, b.1914, integrated Sivananda with the Integral Yoga tradition founded by Sri Auribindo.

RENAISSANCE OF HINDUISM & HATHA YOGA FROM 1850 ONWARD:

INTEGRAL YOGA

SIKHISM.
15TH CENTURY

Practiced by siddha yogis, who combined the search for enlightenment with the perfecting of paranormal powers through Tantrism.

Mira Richard

Disciple of Sri Auribindo Ghosh.

Sri Auribindo Ghosh
1872–1950

Founded Pondicherry Ashram in India in 1914.

SIVANANDA

HATHA YOGA
C. 900 C.E.

By the 1300s texts on Hatha Yoga, most notably the Hatha Yoga Pradipika, were established. They were effectively the first yoga manuals, covering asana, pranayama, bandha and cleansing practices.

BIKRAM YOGA

Bishnu Gosh
1902–1970

Brother of Pramahansa Yogananda.

Swami Vishnu Devananda

Arrived in Montreal in 1957. Established the Sivananda Yoga Vendanta Centers all over the world.

TANTRISM
C. 500–1000 C.E.

Bikram Choudry
b.1945

Deepak Chopra

Became a guru in his own right, encouraged to take the spiritual path by Maharishi Mahesh Yogi

SHANKARA
C. 800 C.E.

Swami Vishvananda

Of Sringen Math.

Swami Sivananada Saraswati
1887–1963

Sent his disciple, Vishnu Devananda, to the West.

PATANJALI AND THE SUTRA PERIOD
C. 200 C.E.

Yoga and other Indian philosophies are organized into identifiable systems and doctrine. Patanjali's system is the classical basis of yoga practice.

Swami Brahmananda Saraswati
d.1993

Formerly known as Ramamurti S. Mishra, M.D., and the founder of the Yoga Society of New York (1958) and San Francisco (1973).

Maharishi Mahesh Yogi
b.1920

Settled in U.S. and founded Transcendental Meditation in 1957

EPIC PERIOD
C. 600 B.C.E.—C.E.

TRANSCENDENTAL MEDITATION

HIMALAYAN INSTITUTE

VEDIC PERIOD
C. 2500–600 B.C.E.

The sacred hymns set the tone for the development of Indian faith and philosophy, both orthodox and unorthodox.

Swami Rama
1925–1996

CIVILIZATION OF THE INDUS VALLEY
C. 4000–2000 B.C.E.

Baba Dharam Das
d.1982

PRE-VEDIC ANIMISM.

BEFORE 4000 B.C.E.

A time when people worshipped natural phenomena and the mother goddess.

THE YOGA GRAPEVINE

YOGA SCHOOLS

SIDDHA YOGA ~ The Siddha Yoga teachings spring from Advaita Vedanta philosophy and the scriptures of Kashmiri Shaivism, as well as the *Bhagavad Gita*. Shaivism is a branch of the Shaivite philosophical tradition based on aphorisms supposed to have been revealed to a ninth-century sage, Vasugupta, by the god Shiva. Siddha means "perfected one."

Siddha Yoga was brought to the West by Swami Muktananda. A wandering sadhu from an early age, he met Guru Bhagwan Nityananda and was inspired to follow his path of Siddha Yoga. Nityananda lived in near-seclusion in southern India and it was he who, in the 1970s, sent Muktananda to the West to teach self-realization through Siddha meditation. Swami Muktananda set up the SYDA foundation in the United States as well as establishing the "mother" ashram of the Siddha Yoga movement, the Gurudev Siddha Peeth, as a public trust in Maharashtra state in India. His protégée, Gurumayi Chidvilasananda, took on his mantle

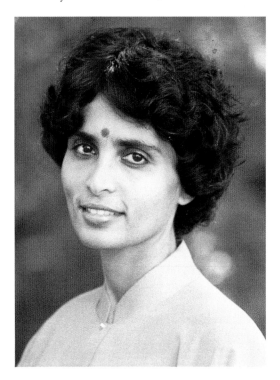

as head of the Siddha Yoga movement after he died, and travels, as did her guru, all over the world teaching the yoga path of enlightenment. She resides at the main U.S. headquarters of the SYDA foundation, the Shree Muktananda Ashram in the Catskill Mountains of New York.

Siddha yogis believe that all religions are equal – that the highest truth is found at the point at which all differences between religions disappear. They teach that we have lost the blissful state of our innately good inner nature, and that this can be restored through the practice of yoga, which centers us and reconnects us with God. The guru's role is to show us the way back into ourselves in order that our potential for enlightenment might be awakened. The emphasis is on *shaktipat*, "spiritual awakening." Students study chanting, contemplation, and the writings of the sages and offer selfless service, under the guidance of a guru, as a means to self-realization. There is also a great emphasis on the power of mantras and the well-being, beauty, and joy that devotional music can inspire.

Today there are hundreds of independently licensed Siddha Yoga Meditation centers all over the world, as well as the two main ashrams in India and New York State. Both have become places of pilgrimage and spiritual retreat where intensive courses on meditation, chanting, and Hatha Yoga are all offered.

IYENGAR YOGA ~ Best known in the United States as the Yogi who established "pretzel yoga," Bellur Krishnamachar Sundararaja Iyengar, now known to his pupils as "Guruji," is the founder of the Iyengar school of yoga and still teaching in his eighties from his base in Pune in southern India. He trained from the age of sixteen with Sri Krishnamacharya. Two years later he left Krishnamacharya and went to teach in Pune. Alone there and far from his guru, he

Yoga teaches us to cure what need not be endured and endure what cannot be cured.
B.K.S. IYENGAR

Left. Is it Gurumayi's extraordinary charisma that has brought her a devoted following of many thousands? She is aware of the tightrope she walks between being a guru on the one hand and a humble disciple on the other.

B.K.S. Iyengar is certainly one of the most influential yoga teachers in the United States, where he has a very strong following.

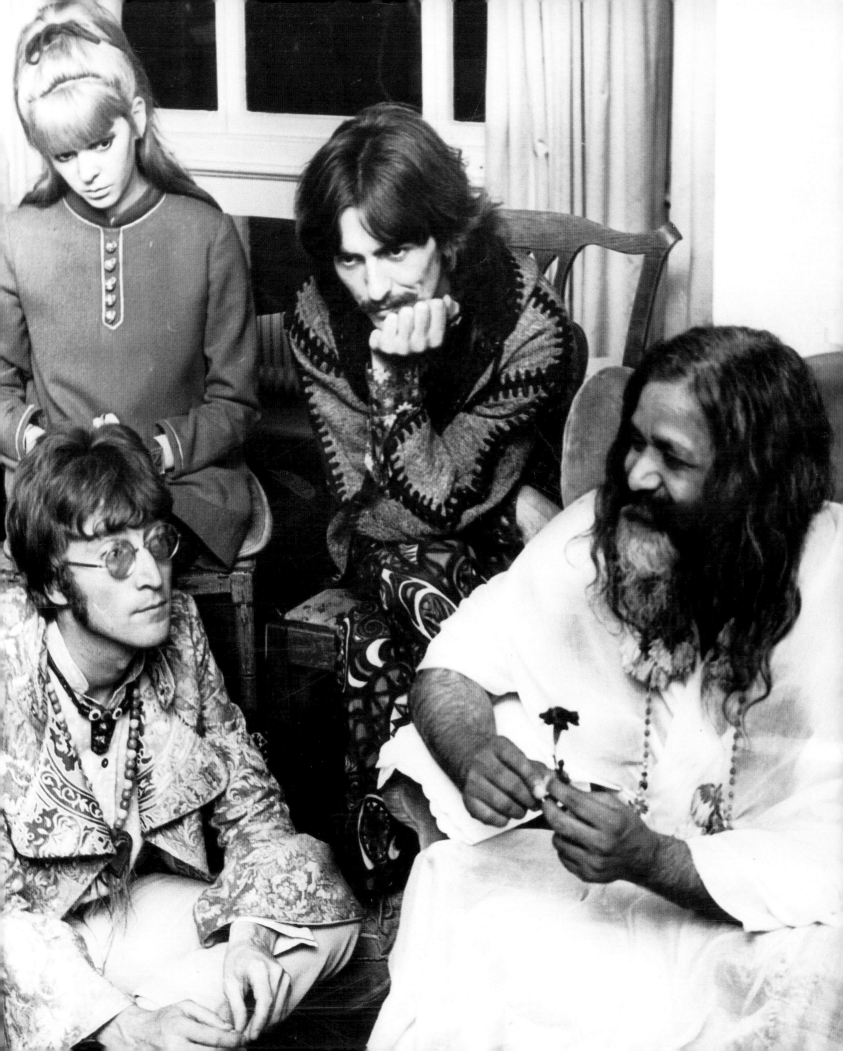

*Left. Maharishi Mahesh
Yogi speaking to John
Lennon, Ringo Starr's
wife Maureen, and
George Harrison, in
about 1967.*

refined his knowledge, technique, and understanding of yoga, although to start with it did not bring him enough money to live on. His arranged marriage to Ramamani, Krishnamacharya's sister, brought him a family, and two of his children teach in his ashram today. Eventually word got out that Iyengar was a great teacher, and he was sought out by luminaries such as Krishnamurti and Jayaprakash Narayan. His meeting with the great violinist Yehudi Menuhin in the 1950s led to a lifelong friendship and to Menuhin's almost evangelical zeal for yoga. Thanks to him, Iyengar came not only to teach in the West but to train others to teach his methods. Eventually, in 1975, he opened what is now the Ramamani Iyengar Memorial Yoga Institute, to cater for the increasing numbers of Westerners wanting to work with him. Now eighty-two years old, Iyengar still attracts pupils. Classes are up to one-hundred strong in Pune and there is a three-year waiting list for students from abroad.

Perhaps Iyengar's greatest influence has been through his book, *Light on Yoga*, first published in 1966. This encyclopedic work has become a classic reference, and inspired and enriched the lives of yoga students worldwide, cutting across gender, religion, caste, and geographical divisions. It is still in print in eighteen languages. There are now more than two hundred centers of Iyengar Yoga across the world, where yoga is taught with their founder's vigorous, analytical approach, emphasizing, particularly at the Pune institute, the practice of yoga as therapy for illness and other physical conditions, and highlighting Iyengar's phenomenal understanding of the body and its self-healing powers.

TRANSCENDENTAL MEDITATION (TM)

~ The Maharishi Mahesh Yogi studied the science of consciousness with his guru, Swami Brahmananda Sarasvati, for thirteen years. He then spent two years in silence in the Himalayas before founding the Transcendental Meditation movement, which teaches a technique now practiced by millions of people all over the world. It is promoted as the simplest and most effective technique for gaining deep relaxation, inner happiness, and fulfillment. And indeed the technique appears to have been validated by research, which includes studies into improved health, cognitive performance, and even reductions in crime rates related to the practice of TM. Several controlled studies have shown that one percent of the population of a community practicing TM or the advanced TM-Sidhi program can lead to a reduction of levels of violence, crime, accident, and disease within that society as a whole. Neuroscience also suggests that meditators who have been practicing TM for more than five years record average levels twelve years younger than their actual age in tests for blood pressure and visual and auditory performance.

The Maharishi can also be credited with promoting the understanding and use of Ayurvedic medicine, the traditional Indian healing system, which was almost unheard of in the West half a century ago and is now a familiar branch of alternative health. Nevertheless, Maharishi Mahesh Yogi's commercial acumen and capacity for self-promotion has brought him his fair share of criticism. He has always acted on a grand scale and is remembered particularly for captivating The Beatles, literally transforming the way they led their lives after they met him. His powerful TM movement proselytizes actively among undergraduate students in universities all over the world, charging not insubstantial sums for initiation into the techniques of TM, and promising better exam results in return. Maharishi Yogi has also turned his interest in Ayurveda into a big business, through his endorsement of a whole range of Ayurvedic medicines.

In 1988 he drafted a masterplan to "Create Heaven on earth for the reconstruction of the whole world inner and outer." The idea was to gather a huge group of many thousands of advanced meditators, whose synchronized influence on the collective consciousness across the planet would neutralize stress and promote world peace. Groups of people still gather on a regular basis to practice TM techniques together with the aim of affecting collective consciousness.

On a smaller scale, practitioners of TM learn to meditate in the standard way taught since Patanjali and before, with a secret mantra given to them at a local TM center. "Transcendental Meditation," says the Maharishi "is not a set of beliefs, a philosophy, a lifestyle, or a religion, it's an experience, a mental technique one practices every day for fifteen or twenty minutes." Like most meditation techniques, TM highlights the importance of the "settled state," one that is neither in the active state of being awake nor in one of the two states of sleep that comprise dreaming and forgetfulness. Once this fourth state of consciousness is accessed, the mind is at its most alert, most creative, and most precise. The combination of the deep relaxation that TM brings and this clarity of mind allows for better physical and mental performance and improved health.

VINIYOGA ~ Krishnamacharya, the father of T.K.V. Desikachar, broke all sorts of social taboos when he opened his yoga school in Mysore in the early 1930s to teach yoga. He was born into a family that traced its roots back to a famous ninth-century sage called Nathamuni, who was the first teacher in the line of Vaishnavite gurus, worshippers of Vishnu – by contrast with Shaivites, those who worship Shiva. He was enrolled at Brahmatantra Parakala Mutt, one of the most

respected Brahmin schools, and studied the Vedic texts from the age of twelve.

In 1916, Krishnamacharya went to the Himalayas where he met his teacher, Sri Ramamohan Brahmachari, a learned yogi who was living in Tibet. Here he learned Ayurveda as well as yoga at its deepest levels. When his seven years with his teacher were up and Krishnamacharya asked how he should pay for his apprenticeship, he was told that he must go back to the world, raise a family, and teach yoga. Such a path was considered well beneath the aspirations of an educated Brahmin and recognized scholar, but Krishnamacharya stayed true to his teacher's command despite great poverty and the incomprehension of his peers, and lived to become one of the fathers of modern yoga, being the teacher of B.K.S. Iyengar, Pattabhi Jois, and Indra Devi, and his own son, T.K.V. Desikachar.

Krishnamacharya was still teaching and healing until six weeks before his death at the age of 101. Desikachar founded the Krishnamacharya Yoga Mandiram in 1976. It is both a teacher training center and an institution for using yoga to treat the sick. It calls its school of yoga "Viniyoga," and puts great emphasis on teaching the individual, with the belief that the teaching of yoga must be tailored to fit the person, not the other way around, and that the yoga path will therefore mean different things to different people: "Yoga for one person can mean becoming healthy again, for another it can mean finding help in preparing for death. For a child it is interesting and meaningful to have a lot of physical exertion – but why should I teach an eighty-year-old person to do a headstand or sit in the lotus position?" said Krishnamacharya.

VANDA SCARAVELLI ~ Vanda Scaravelli was in the privileged position of being able to afford to follow many yoga gurus. She was a close friend of

"It is not so much the performance of the exercises that matters, but rather the way we are doing them." Vanda Scaravelli and Mary Stewart discuss just this *"doing of them"* with all the animation and intelligence that both have brought to their teaching.

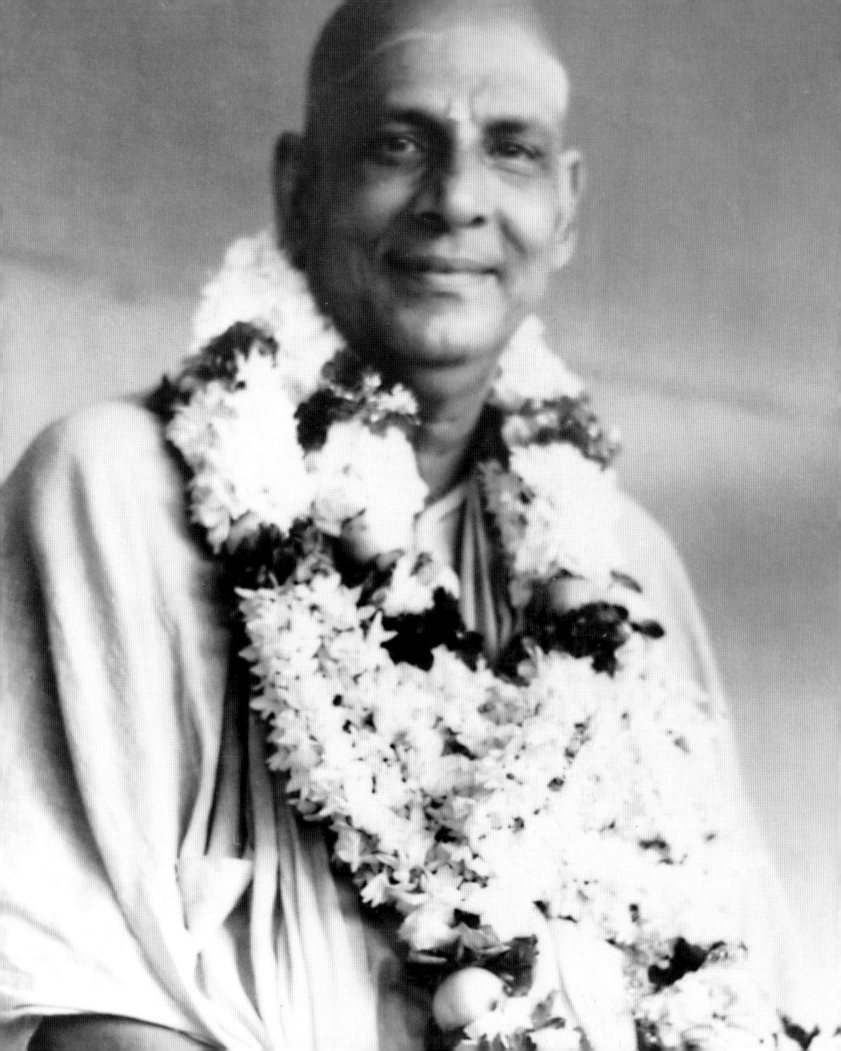

Krishnamurti, became a pupil of Iyengar, and later met and worked with Desikachar and many other luminaries of the yoga world in Canada, England, Italy, and Switzerland. She went on to develop her own technique of yoga, which owes much more to breathing and the "song of the body" than most other systems. Her friend and collaborator, Iyengar-trained Mary Stewart, worked with her in developing this system that has spawned a gentler, more fluid yoga, which is about real grounding, both mental and physical, and the release of energy that comes from it. Scaravelli's book, *Awakening the Spine*, has become required reading, but she always adamantly refused to give her name to a school of yoga. Nevertheless, many of the second and third generations of those who were influenced by her identify the sort of yoga they practice and teach with her name, and since her death in 1999, there has been little anyone can do about that.

SIVANANDA YOGA ~ Swami Sivananda Saraswati (1887–1963) was born in Tamil Nadu in southern India. He became a doctor of medicine in Malaysia, but in 1923 he was called by God, renounced the world, and left everything to settle in the Himalayas for seven years of meditation. In 1936 he founded The Divine Life Society, and twelve years later the Sivananda Ashram and the Yoga Vedanta Forest Academy. In 1957 he sent his disciple Swami Vishnu Devananda to the West with the words "many souls in the East are reincarnating in the West. Go and reawaken their consciousness and bring them back to the path of yoga."

Swami Vishnu Devananda then traveled through North America teaching yoga and observing the Western lifestyle. He established the first headquarters of the Sivananda Centre in Montreal in 1961 and the first Yoga camp in Val Morin, Quebec, in 1962. Now there are ashrams in Kerala in southern India, America, Canada, the

An ounce of practice is worth ten tons of theory.
SWAMI VISHNU DEVANANDA

Left. Swami Sivananda, founder of the Sivananda school of yoga.

Bahamas and the Himalayas, as well as centers in the United Kingdom, Europe, Israel, and Uruguay.

Sivananda Yoga is based on the Gurukula system – *guru* means teacher and *kula* means home. Students would arrive at the ashram at the age of eight and remain for twelve years, during which time they would study philosophy, as well as asanas, pranayama, and Karma Yoga. Today the yoga courses are based on this model: For an intensive four-week program you live, study, and work with teachers and students, wear a uniform and live in the ashram environment. The diet is vegetarian and the emphasis is on a rounded life of exercise, proper breathing, relaxation, positive thinking, and meditation. This is very much along the lines of the classical Vedanta teaching, and would seem profoundly rigorous were it not for the fact that one can become a Sivananda yoga teacher after only four weeks of teacher-training.

Unlike some yoga classes, the Sivananda regimen involves one program of twelve basic asanas, with the addition of Salute to the Sun and starting with Headstand, and uses it repeatedly. The sequence of asanas covers all the movements required for health and well-being, but for the average undisciplined Western body, this is quite hard core. Talk of opening up chakras begins in the most elementary classes. Interestingly, a high level of execution of advanced asanas is becoming part of the modern approach to yoga in the West, very much through the influence of Sivananda.

BIKRAM YOGA ~ Bikram Choudry was born in 1945. His guru was Bishnu Ghosh, the brother of Paramahansa Yogananda who wrote *Autobiography of a Yogi*. At the age of twelve he was the National Yoga Champion of India. At twenty he was told he would never walk again after a weight-lifting accident. He created his series of yoga postures to restore his own health and now teaches it to others. What particularly distinguishes this from other yoga systems is that the poses are physically extremely demanding and are practiced in a heated room so that muscles, ligaments, and joints can stretch further and without injury. The heated environment also promotes profuse sweating, which helps flush toxins from the body. For a time, Bikram lived in London teaching at the Yoga College of India, but in the eighties he moved on to a rather more glamorous existence in Beverly Hills, and has opened three centers of his own in New York City in the last couple of years, which are said to attract large numbers of dancers, actors, and other body workers.

KUNDALINI YOGA ~ Sri Singh Sahib Bhai Sahib Harbhajan Singh Khalsa Yogiji, otherwise known as Yogi Bhajan, founded the "3HO," the Healthy Happy Holy Foundation, in 1969. Also called the "Yoga of Awareness," the yoga it teaches is commonly referred to as Kundalini yoga, although it does not concentrate particularly on the raising of the kundalini, but promises "to help you be the best you can be." The 3HO is now a training organization with centers all over the world.

Born in what is now Pakistan, Yogi Bhajan was the son of a Sikh doctor, and mastered Kundalini yoga when he was sixteen. When India was partitioned in 1947 he took charge of leading a thousand people out of his village to safety in New Delhi. During his youth he studied with many teachers, including his grandfather and the Mahan Tantric, Sant Hazara Singh. Married with three children, he was a commanding officer in the Indian Army and served in the Indian Government for eighteen years before he moved to America.

Many of Yogi Bhajan's followers have become Sikhs. (The first Sikh leader was Guru Nanak, who died in 1539. His followers were called Sishyas or Sikhs, which translates as "students.") Yogi Bhajan calls his Kundalini yoga a "creative catalyst,"

a technology that gets the best out of people. Kundalini teachers give classes that include asanas that are familiar and rooted in classical Indian yoga but have a distinctly Western flavor. The poses are devised to stimulate organs, develop a healthy body and emotional balance, and aim to bring about enlightenment, in much the same way as other schools, but they have been developed particularly for an American audience, even though there are now more than three hundred centers teaching this method in thirty-five countries. One of the best-known Kundalini teachers after Yogi Bhajan, Gurmukh, has written her own book and is known in Los Angeles for her celebrity clientele.

ASHTANGA YOGA ~ Ashtanga Yoga is named after the practice of yoga as laid down by the sage, Patanjali. In his Yoga Sutras, he talks of the ashtanga path, *ashta* meaning eight and *anga* meaning limb. Most schools of yoga take Patanjali's eightfold path as their basis, but there is now also a school of yoga called Ashtanga yoga, with a very particular emphasis. The most high profile of the proponents of Ashtanga yoga is Pattabhi Jois, who was a student of Krishnamacharya. In 1948 Jois founded the Ashtanga Yoga Institute in Mysore, where he developed a series of poses "based on purifying practices described in the ancient texts." It is a fast-paced, gymnastic type of yoga, which has become very popular in the West, most probably because it represents the smallest shift from gym-culture to yoga. Much emphasis is placed on energizing postures which are challenging for the beginner and for the stiff Western body. Students jump into the postures and jump back with a lot of aerobic activity that does not form a part of other yoga systems. Many people start Ashtanga Yoga as an alternative to working out in the gym and then surprise themselves with the discovery that the yoga

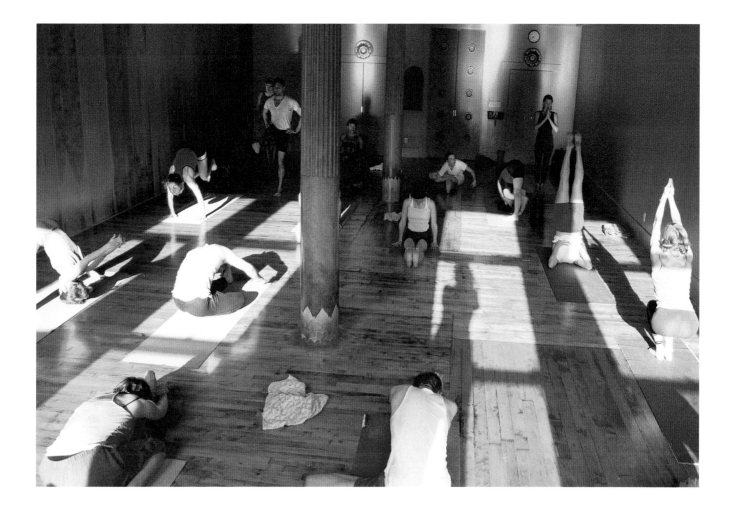

is influencing their daily lives in a more profound way than the gym ever did. From there some become interested in the quieter, more meditative aspects of yoga.

The Ashtanga Yoga taught by Baba Hari Dass in California is an altogether more classical affair, with the flavor of the sort of yoga preferred in the 1960s and 1970s.

"HATHA FUSION" ~ One significant development of the new wave of yoga in Europe and the United States is that many yoga centers are opening up with several different types of yoga offered. Meanwhile, as workshops and training courses abound, more and more of the new generation of yoga teachers are taking their influence from several different sources, combining the ideas and approaches that suit them, and making it increasingly difficult to identify which school they come from. This is a healthy sign, an acknowledgment that teachers cannot be clones of their gurus, and that every individual will bring a personal own element to his or her teaching. With today's obsession for labels, some people call this "Hatha Fusion," but this amounts to little more than an acknowledgment that teaching evolves in its own way from one generation to the next.

The Tao of nurturing life requires that one keep oneself as fluid and flexible as possible. One should not stay still for too long, nor should one exhaust oneself by trying to perform impossible tasks. One should learn how to exercise from nature by observing the fact that flowing water never stagnates and a busy door with active hinges never rusts or rots. Why? Because they exercise themselves perpetually and are almost always moving.

SUN SSU-MO, TANG DYNASTY PHYSICIAN

THE PRACTICE OF YOGA could easily be presented in twenty-first-century marketing terms as the ultimate health and beauty device. It now often enjoys the endorsement of conventional medicine, as it has proved to have beneficial effects in all sorts of areas. But independent of the grudging blessing of the medical profession (which has been a long time coming), one comes to understand more about the body's own incredible potential for self-healing through yoga practice. The body is a miracle of bio-engineering, able to heal wounds, mend bones, fight infection, restore depleted energy, and resist all kinds of virus. Nevertheless, contemporary Western life has largely ignored this capacity for vital health, preferring an existence with little exercise or nourishing food, and popping what it assumes will be instant cures in the form of pills and prescriptions when problems arise.

The most immediately apparent way in which the practice of yoga asanas helps the body is in improving the flexibility and mobility of the spine and joints. Many people take up yoga in the first place as a result of injury or immobility, because yoga inflicts a very low level of impact on the body while giving it an all-over stretch and tone. Traditionally, yoga was practiced almost entirely by men. However, when it first came to the West, it tended to be women who took it up, men feeling it was slightly effeminate and rather too alternative. This has changed considerably in the past decade, since hardcore calisthenics and a Herculean standard of competition in athletic fields has led quite often to permanent physical damage. While it's not clear how many athletes would admit to doing full-fledged yoga, there are few who do not now practice yoga-based exercises as a part of their daily routine.

At the other end of the spectrum, in the context of modern living, where there is too much sitting on comfortable chairs and being driven to and from destinations, the gentle and thoughtful stretching and bending of the body into yoga asanas has proved to be a totally safe form of exercise.

Another general way in which yoga promotes health is through the positive influence the asanas have on the circulation of the blood. With the therapeutic twists and turns of the body and the controled breathing, blood pulses through those parts of the body where it can have a tendency to be sluggish. This in turn raises the level of oxygen distribution around the system and aids the removal of toxins. People who practice yoga regularly find that their immune systems are stronger, they get fewer chronic complaints such as colds, ear infections, and other minor aches and pains, and have better circulation, better skin tone, and more energy. They are usually surprised and delighted by this, but there is more. The internal organs are toned and massaged by specific postures. Take the abdominal twists that, as the spine corkscrews, give a gentle massage to the liver and kidneys, or the Shoulderstand, in which gentle pressure is put on the shoulders and neck, stimulating the thyroid gland. The careful use of these postures means that a rich diet and stressful working life can be relieved, not with drugs and stimulants but with the disciplined practice of yogic asanas.

As well as all this, asanas and pranayama exert a powerful, albeit subtle, influence on the nervous system, most particularly through the careful lengthening and stimulation of the spine in almost every pose. Meanwhile, deep breathing and meditation have proved to slow down the heart rate, lower the blood pressure and alleviate stress.

Very occasionally, breathing and postures can have immediate results. It is not uncommon for people to burst into tears in the middle of a yoga class because some deep-seated tension held somewhere in their bodies has been released. However, this is not the norm. The results of yoga come from a slow, gentle, committed process of daily practice. It takes time to unlock long-term muscular tightness and distortion, bad postural habits, and the tendencies of a stressful and nervous existence, and it takes time to cure oneself completely of addictions and habits, whether physical or mental. This is why yoga has never been a quick fix route to thin thighs, athletic prowess, and a calm persona, although all of these do come eventually.

Right. Preparation for Virabhadrasana, or Warrior pose, which is named after Virabhadra, a warrior hero created by Shiva, chief of the gods. The great fighter is both strong and controlled, and Warrior pose demands vigor and balance.

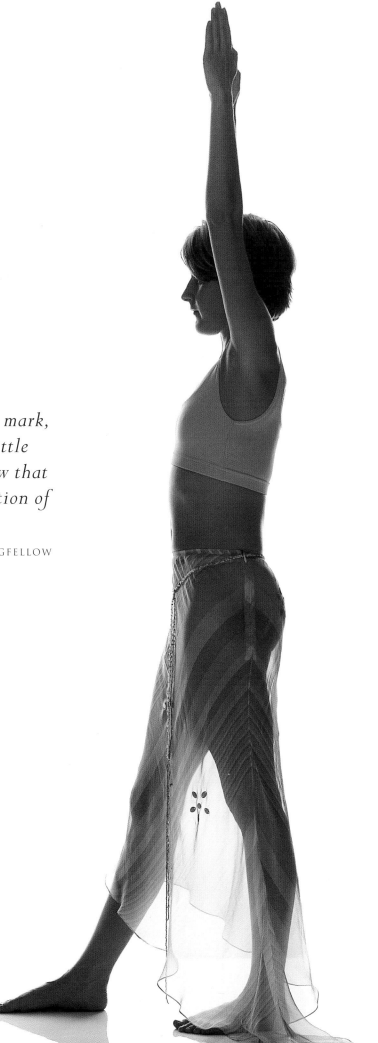

*If you would hit the mark,
you must aim a little
above it; Every arrow that
flies feels the attraction of
the earth.*

"ELEGIAC VERSE," H.W. LONGFELLOW

DIET FOR LIFE

One of the by-products of practicing yoga is an instinctive desire to complement the good you are doing to your body with a better diet. Almost without being aware of it, people who've been practicing yoga for a while begin to change their diets and eat the food that we all now know to be good for us; a large proportion of raw or lightly steamed vegetables, fruit and grains, nuts, seeds, and smaller amounts of dairy products and meat – all without preservatives or artificial flavorings. There are all kinds of theories about what yogis should and should not eat. However, it is important to be intelligent about this. The ideal diet in a country like India is a vegetarian one and the whole Ayurvedic system of medicine is based on this. But for those who do not live in the culture or climate of the East, other considerations must be taken into account. In colder climates and for those with low blood pressure, a vegetarian diet might not be entirely suitable. Meanwhile, and luckily for the Beverly Hills set of yoga devotees, experts haven't decided yet whether a glass or two of wine is damaging or actually good for you.

The science of yoga holds that the mind is formed from the essence of the food we eat. And on the balance of the three characteristics of all matter – the *gunas*: *tamas*, putrified or inert; *rajas*, stimulating or active; and *sattva*, pure – the yogi should stick to a diet that is based on sattvic foods. But we mustn't forget that these three gunas make up the universe in yogic cosmology, and all three are required in the correct balance if both the macro universe of the cosmos and the micro universe of our bodies are to function properly.

The guidelines for healthy eating are laid out in the *Bhagavad Gita*. The three elements divide roughly as follows.

Sattvic foods are fresh and untampered with. They consist of grains and unpolished rice, protein in the form of nuts and seeds, and fruits both fresh and dried. Such foods encourage life, purity, strength, health, cheerfulness, and calm.

Rajasic foods are bitter, sour, salty, hot and spicy, pungent, dry, and burning. Tea, coffee, caffeinated drinks, salty snacks, chemical-ridden convenience foods, tobacco, and stimulants of all kinds fall into this category. They are considered to be over-stimulating to the mind as well as irritating to the mucous membrane of the intestines.

Tamasic foods are all foods that are stale or overripe. This covers all meat, alcohol, and other fermented food, all narcotics such as hashish and opium, and food that has been deep-fried or reheated. Tamasic food makes a person lazy and dull and it accentuates a tendency to suffer from chronic ailments.

Doctors now acknowledge that a poor diet can be responsible for a sluggish immune system and that a good diet can go a long way toward treating many forms of disease. The discipline of yoga works in tandem with a better diet, and the two together can help to break compulsive habits and patterns of behavior. All the stresses of a modern lifestyle can be eased with specific poses, and in many cases the great yoga teachers have developed programs of postures and breathing combined with strict diets to cure all manner of ailments. Desikachar opened his Krishnamacharaya Yoga Mandiram in order to treat the sick through yoga, much of the teaching of B.K.S. Iyengar is based on its therapeutic properties, while the Maharishi Mahesh Yogi has concentrated on health through breathing, meditation, and an Ayurvedic diet. They have all written books with detailed and instructive chapters on which postures they recommend to treat specific problems.

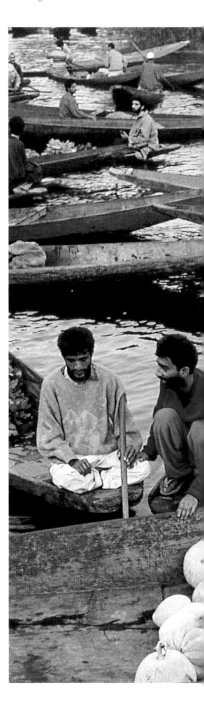

The true yogi knows that you are what you eat, never neglecting his or her body and eating, always in moderation, the freshest sattvic foods.

On a personal note, I have watched in classes over the years the stiffest, most arthritic yoga practitioners gain mobility they never dreamed of; and, in one instance, a woman who had had a brain tumor removed from one side of her head, work slowly and surely, against the predictions of her doctors, until she could do all sorts of advanced yoga positions and had regained complete mobility, health, and quality of life.

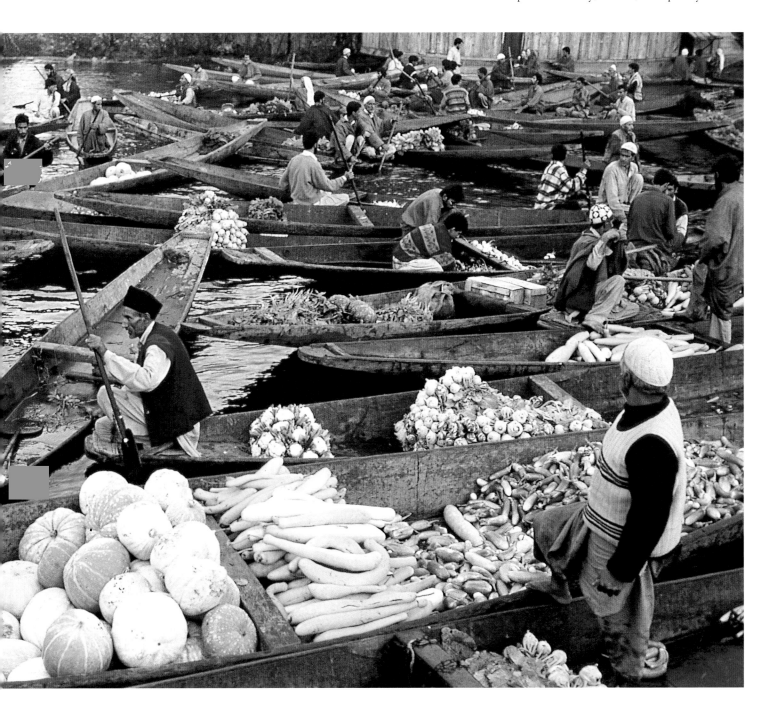

ASANAS FOR AILMENTS

Always consult a doctor before you start – get a qualified opinion and be intelligent about what you do. Your body is not like any other and it will not react in exactly the same way as another. More important, it's the only one you have, so look after it. Don't expect instant results, and don't overdo a pose that works at the expense of a balanced practice, or you'll start having problems somewhere else in your body. Finally, there is no point in doing yoga postures for a complaint if you are then going to go and pound your body in the gym as well.

Not all of the poses listed below are demonstrated in this book, as it does not set out to be a manual – refer to any good yoga manual for those you cannot find here.

ADDICTION ~ This is not one to tackle alone. Get a good, patient teacher and backup from Alcoholics Anonymous or Narcotics Anonymous. You should concentrate on standing poses – but not those requiring balancing on one leg – and Headstand and Shoulderstand. Avoid backbends and intense breathing exercises.

BACKACHE ~ Lie flat on the floor with your legs bent up and give time to just breathe and relax. Put cushions under your head or legs up onto a chair. All standing poses except the twists – such as Triangle – can help; Tree, Forward Bend onto a table, Warrior, and eventually a Shoulderstand with the help of a chair or wall.

CONSTIPATION ~ Over-prepared and over-refined foods combined with stress and lack of exercise often leads to constipation, which itself holds toxins in the body and undermines the whole system. Several cycles of Salute to the Sun can deal with constipation very effectively. Failing that, try lots of Shoulderstand variations and Plough.

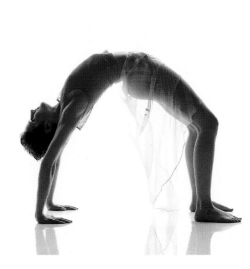

The intense stretch of the spine and opening up of the chest in Backbend is a wonderful antidote to depression.

DEPRESSION ~ Start working on sitting up straight with your shoulders dropped. All the Standing poses give energy and vitality; Salute to the Sun, Headstand, and backbends are helpful, too. As for breathing, do Simhasana, Kappalabhati, Kumbaka, and Bramari breathing.

EYE STRAIN ~ Staring at computers and television screens is a constant strain on the eyes. To relax them there is nothing better than lying with a compress or rice bag across the eyes, the gentle, even weight of which releases the tensions of the frown, keeps the eyes closed, and blocks out all light. Sanmukhi mudra is also invaluable for strained eyes. Sit in lotus and close your eyes. Then put your hands softly onto your face, thumbs in your ears, index fingers on your eyebrows, middle fingers just below your eyes, the ring finger at the corners of your nostrils and the little fingers at the corners of your mouth. Exhale as the pressure of the fingers gently widens your face. If your eyes are badly strained, it may not be a good idea to do Headstand or other inverted poses.

HEADACHE ~ Regular practice of Shoulderstand helps to prevent headaches and migraines, but don't do it when you actually have a headache. Twists are very helpful, too, either the supine twist, lying on the back, or any of the sitting twists.

HIPS ~ Stiff hips can cause bad backs. Try Cobblers pose and sit there for some time, leaning against a wall if necessary. Kneeling poses, like Vajrasana, and inverted poses, in which the hips can be worked without any weight on them, can be particularly helpful for arthritic hips.

Many chronic knee problems can be addressed simply by learning to stand quietly and evenly on both feet.

KNEE PROBLEMS ~ Inverted poses are wonderful for the knees because the joints can be worked without bearing any weight. Also give a lot of time to Mountain pose, learning how to stand firm and quiet and even on your feet. Sitting up straight with the legs wide apart in a pose called Upavista Konasana is also good for feeling the backs of the knees open without hyperextension.

SHOULDERS AND NECK ~ Everyday use of computers, telephones, cars, and the pace and stresses of daily life cause most people to hold a lot of their tension in their neck and shoulders. Usually one side is worse than the other, so work more on the stiffer one. Cow pose, Eagle pose, Triangle, supine twists, Forward bend onto a chair or, if you are flexible, as far as your toes, Child's pose, Dog, Locust, and Sitting Forward bend are all good for this. Tight shoulder and neck muscles can contribute to headaches.

STRESS ~ Lie as for backache, breathing gently with the whole spine long and flat on the floor, for at least five minutes. When your breathing is slow and regular, gently fold in your knees and hug them to you without tightening your shoulders. Child's pose is a fabulous one for stress, as are the shoulder releases like Cow and Eagle arms. If you are

turning this into a full practice, move on to standing poses, Shoulderstand, and then the supine twists. Leave plenty of time at the end for a long Savasana, or Corpse pose.

VARICOSE VEINS ~ Headstand and Shoulderstand, and all the variations of these that you can do.

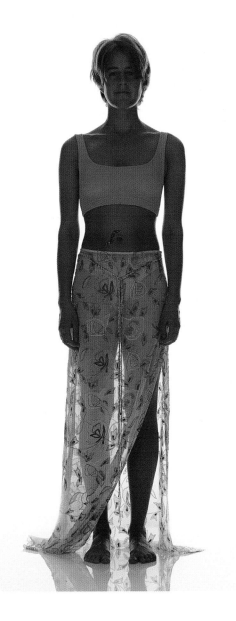

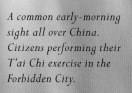

A common early-morning sight all over China. Citizens performing their T'ai Chi exercise in the Forbidden City.

Yoga has close connections with other ancient forms of exercise, and has formed the basis of many more modern exercise systems as well. The martial arts, for example, derived from the yoga asanas and pranayama that arrived in China in the fifth century. This introduction is attributed to the Buddhist monk, Bodhidharma. The fusion of his yoga teaching with the indigenous Chinese system Dao-Yin resulted in what we know today as martial arts. What is so easily forgotten about the martial arts is that they were conceived as a means of fighting disease, not as a means of fighting the enemy. In all ancient cultures exercise was a compliment to medicine, the way toward holistic health and the strength that comes from physical well-being. The Chinese view their popular systems, T'ai Chi, Qi Gong, and Wing Chun, as exercises that focus the mind and develop inner strength. The latest thinking on diet and exercise has come into line with these doctrines. Now sports and medical bodies assert that moderate physical exercise is far better for body and mind than quick-fix over-exertion. All top athletes are learning that heavy cardiovascular exercise without the contrasting stretch, relax, and breathe element results in burnout and injury. For most people it is regular, moderate exercise that will provide a stronger immune system, as well as renewed energy and balance. Over centuries, bits and pieces of different exercise systems have crossed cultures and hemispheres, been taught and reworked, assimilated by new disciples, and given new names. It is striking how many of today's popular fitness options – both in the bodily positions and in the breathing instruction – owe something to yoga, the oldest system of them all.

ECHOES OF YOGA

T'AI CHI ~ T'ai Chi involves the co-ordination of body, breath, and balance with the aim of harmonizing essence, energy and spirit. In China people practice in parks and offices at sunrise, for according to Chinese philosophy this is when nature's *chi* or vital energy, flows most strongly. T'ai Chi is a sort of meditation in motion, which involves a series of movements, each called a form. The forms are performed slowly, fluidly, continuously, one after the other, with the weight very solidly grounded in the feet so that the chi of the practitioner can move freely from the centered starting point. As in yoga, the movements have names taken from nature – Eagle, Monkey, Cobra Unwinds, and so on. It looks easy when done well but it requires strength and precision. In China it is done by the old and the young alike, as it benefits both mind and body, promoting self-control and concentration as well as being good for the blood circulation, for strengthening the lower back, and for improving the functioning of the internal and respiratory organs.

QI GONG ~ Qi Gong is about energy cultivation and, along with acupuncture and herbalism, is one of the bases of traditional Chinese medicine since it was first practiced by Chinese doctors. The movements are small and performed slowly. Qi Gong means "the curing of illness through muscle movement." As with T'ai Chi and yoga, there are several systems of Qi Gong (pronounced "chi gung") in China, where it is apparently practiced by around sixty million people.

THE ALEXANDER TECHNIQUE ~ Frederick Matthias Alexander was an Australian who developed his system at the beginning of the twentieth century. It is not, as is often thought, a set of exercises to help posture, but a system for releasing unnecessary tension and bad postural habits by consciously controlling the way our bodies work in unison with how we feel. Alexander was actually trying to solve his own throat problems. He noticed by observing how he held himself when he looked in the mirror that he was standing and moving his body in ways of which he was unaware. He found that when the neck became free, the head could come forward and up and his spine could lengthen. By focusing on whether or not he stiffened his neck and hunched his shoulders as he breathed in, he taught himself to stand and move more fluidly. It sounds simplistic, but by working his body and breathing with meticulous attention, he found his whole health improved, including the chronic asthma that had afflicted him since birth. The Alexander Technique is now taught all over the world, and used particularly by drama, art, and music students aiming to reeducate the senses. As with yoga, many people come to it because of injury or back pain and then find it addressing far more than their initial problem, as their whole outlook on life and general health begin to improve. Alexander was persuaded to come to London from Australia in 1904, where he set up a clinic in order to bring the technique to a wider audience. It is unlikely that he was not aware of the theories of the Theosophists at this time or the increased interest in yoga that had arisen in some parts of the world when he was developing his ideas, especially since he taught a number of famous intellectuals connected with the Theosophist movement, including Aldous Huxley and George Bernard Shaw.

PILATES ~ Josef Pilates was born in Dusseldorf, Germany, in 1880. A frail, sickly child, he became obsessed with physical fitness, taking up diving, skiing, boxing, and wrestling to improve his body image. During World War I, he found himself interned in England and spent time devising a fitness program for his fellow internees. After the war, he left Germany for America and set up a studio in New York where some of his earliest disciples were dancers. The late Martha Graham was a devotee. Today a host of A-list celebrities, film stars, models, and dancers are among the millions who have found this system to work for them. They claim it gives them firmer muscles, a leaner frame, better posture, flexibility, and even an increased libido. Pilates involves a series of very controlled, minute, slow, and concentrated movements – there are five hundred in all – performed on a mat and with the help of a spring resistance machine called, rather chillingly, the "reformer." These exercises, linked to the practitioner's center of gravity, lengthen and strengthen the muscles group by group, and involve concentration and great focus. According to its disciples, Pilates's involvement of both mind and body is a key part of its attraction.

FELDENKRAIS ~ For some people even the simplest yoga movements seem both complicated and frightening. For the very unsupple, the idea of contorting the body into what seem to be impossible shapes is more than they can deal with. Moshe Feldenkrais, who died in 1984, founded a system of exercises for just this type of person, as well as for rehabilitation after serious illness. He understood that one could educate the body in a profound way, through even the slowest, smallest, and most subtle movement – if one did it with great concentration and awareness of what the body was doing and how it was responding to the movement. Of course these movements had to be in tune with the anatomy and structure of the body, and Feldenkrais applied his background in physics and engineering to the study of human movement as he developed his system. As with many of the pioneers of contemporary exercise systems, he started with his own chronic knee problem, designing simple floor exercises and bodywork to retrain the central nervous system and unlock stiffness. Feldenkrais can be applied to help in the rehabilitation of trauma, cerebral palsy, and stroke victims. The key aim is body and sensory awareness, and it is impressive how these small, slow movements can release physical tension, letting in flexibility. Yoga practitioners recognize many of the basics of yoga in Feldenkrais, and it can be combined very successfully with yoga postures, especially for stiff and fearful beginners.

To understand others is to have knowledge;
To understand oneself is to be enlightened.
To conquer others requires strength;
To conquer oneself is even harder.
LAO TZE

PRACTICING YOGA

The practice of yoga induces a primary sense of measure and proportion.
Reduced to our own body, our first instrument, we learn to play it, drawing from it maximum resonance and harmony.

YEHUDI MENUHIN

FOR MOST PEOPLE, yoga is the practice of body postures, called asanas, combined with controlled breathing, or pranayama. Asanas and pranayama constitute numbers three and four of the eight limbs or stages of yoga defined by Patanjali. Although they were not devised to show off how to wrap the body into pretzel-like distortions or to raise the heart rate, to the purist, when practiced without the other seven disciplines of yoga, the asanas become little more than a fitness drill. Nevertheless, the practice of asanas is the aspect that most yoga-minded people in the West are interested in. And they have proved to be a remarkably effective antidote to the stress of a high-octane Western lifestyle. Without involving mechanical (and boring) repetition, the asanas are designed to prime every muscle, nerve, and gland in the body, and each pose has its specific function. So, daily practice brings about physical stability, balance, agility, and stamina, as well as mental equilibrium and confidence, a combination that is rarely achieved through dance, athletics, body building, team sports, or any other form of exercise where competition and performance are part of the package.

The word *asana* translates as "posture" from the Sanskrit *as*, which means "to stay," "to be," "to sit." Asanas are the physical exercises that were developed alongside the whole philosophy of yoga in order to keep the body healthy and strong and, as their name suggests, to bring about the more balanced state of mind that comes from giving time just to be.

ASANAS

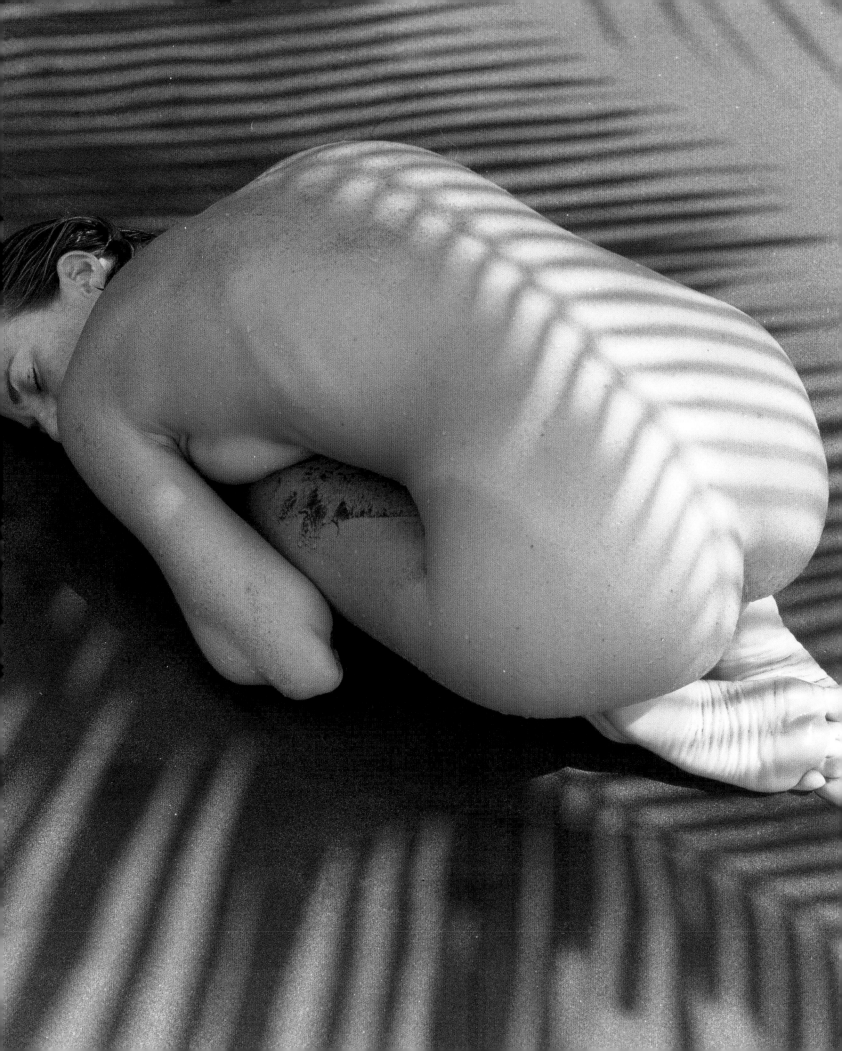

HOW ASANAS WORK

~ Asanas are always performed with a conscious awareness of the breath. The physical action of the breath on the body is an essential component of every asana movement. This conscious link between the postures and the breath is vital also because of the inevitable connection between our physical and emotional selves. Think of how we tense with fear and shake with laughter, and consider the immediate physical effect of these emotional reactions. Because our feelings and emotions are expressed in the way we breathe, any change of mood becomes apparent in how we arrange and move our hands, shoulders, neck, head, and legs. Our disposition will be evident in the way we do the poses, and by the same token, in doing the poses we can learn more about how we are feeling. While the practice of asanas can restore energy, de-stress, and keep the body healthy, their principal importance lies in the way they establish a balance and harmony in the mind and body. A strong, healthy body is one step toward clear-thinking and, ultimately, enlightenment.

All sanity depends on this: that it should be a delight to feel heat strike the skin, a delight to stand upright, knowing the bones are moving easily under the flesh.
DORIS LESSING

Yoga asanas comprise an approach to exercise that is diametrically opposed to the Western approach. Asanas loosen, stretch, and relax the body, while Western exercises tighten and compact it. Yoga postures (like other Eastern forms of exercise including T'ai Chi, Dao-yin, and the martial arts) are slow and rhythmical; Western forms are fast and mechanical. The Western theory of aerobic exercise suggests that you need to pump the heart hard by running and jumping in order to build up strength. In reality you can deplete your energy this way and end up feeling wiped out. Tense spinal muscles block nerve and energy channels and deplete energy by using it up to keep the muscles tight. Eastern regimens aim to undo the stiffness and tensions of the body in order to stretch further, collecting and storing energy in the process and leaving one feeling refreshed. By insisting on movement in harmony with carefully regulated breathing, yoga asanas ensure that, however quiet and subtle the movement, the cardiovascular system is massaged, the bloodstream is oxygenated, and the spine lengthens and stretches, restoring the nerve and energy impulses to the vital organs.

There are three fundamental principles that lie at the heart of every asana. First we must feel grounded by establishing a conscious relationship with how and where gravity is acting on the body; then we bring our attention to the breath, which will settle us in our position and reinforce the connection with the ground. When these first two principles are applied together, the body can begin to release and lengthen, which is the third principle of asana practice.

GRAVITY ~ Gravity pulls against us day in, day out, slowly but surely encouraging us to slump, restricting the movement of our spines and making us shorter as we get older. And yet most of us find it nearly impossible to trust the ground enough to let go and establish a really firm connection with the floor.

THE BREATH ~ One of the reasons for this reluctance to let go is that we have forgotten how to breathe properly. If we lie on our back and make just one really slow, deep breath in and out, most of us can feel how tensions in our body fall away into the floor. This release happens because we have fully engaged the thick band of muscle, the diaphragm, which lies across the bottom of our ribcage and is also attached to the iliopsoas muscles, which are in turn attached to the lumbar vertebrae. When the diaphragm releases with the out breath, the spinal muscles at the back of the waist release, drawing the lower vertebrae down and allowing for the upper vertebrae to lengthen away from them.

LENGTHENING ~ What yoga teaches us is that if we can be aware of our base, the point where gravity is pulling us into the ground, and at the same time conscious of breathing deep in our belly by engaging the diaphragm as we breathe, we can use the pull of gravity as the anchor from which the spine can lengthen and grow upward. Think of a tree or plant whose roots dig deeper and deeper down into the ground in order for the stem, trunk, and branches to grow up to the light and bud and flower. With a conscious awareness of the action of gravity and our breath, we, too, can establish roots and learn to grow.

THE SPINE ~ In the process of learning to root in order to stretch up toward the heavens, the stem, trunk, or spine becomes strong and flexible. In all vertebrates, the spine is the basic support of the body – its structural and neurological core. The spinal cord runs from the brain to the top of the lumbar vertebrae. It is the central axis of the body and the main pathway of the nervous system. Everything about our bodily functions and our movement depends on the health of these nerves. The spinal cord is protected by the vertebrae, which are in turn controlled by layers of muscles and ligaments running up and down the length of the spine, governing posture and movement. To have perfect posture, your head must balance effortlessly at the top of your neck and over the four curves of the spine, and as you move the whole spinal column adjusts and adapts using its proprioceptive sense, in conjunction with all the outer senses, as a guide. Over time and with bad habits, the postural perfection we are born with becomes distorted and we have to unravel the distortions and tensions in order to be in a state of balance. The practice of asanas using the principles described above involves the lengthening and strengthening of these muscles, counteracting the compression of the cartilaginous discs, which makes people shrink with age and is a contributing factor to osteoporosis.

The body is the discipline, the pattern, the law; the spirit is inner devotion, spontaneity, freedom. A body without a spirit is a corpse, and a spirit without a body is a ghost.
RABBI ABRAHAM
JOSHUA HESCHEL

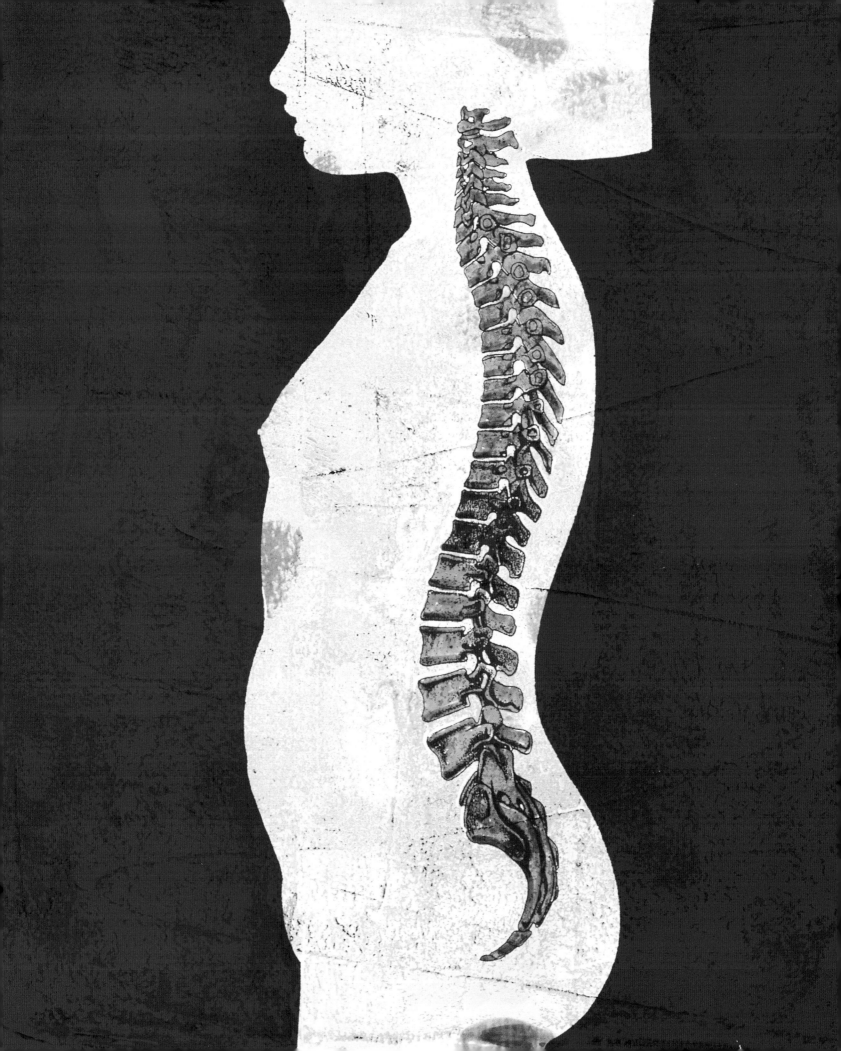

GUIDELINES FOR SAFE PRACTICE ~ When we do yoga asanas, the same postural balance is important whether we are standing, sitting, or upside down. We find this balance, not by gripping and pulling and pushing the body into positions, but by finding our roots – when we are standing our roots are our heels, when upside down they are our elbows or hands, and when sitting they are our two sitting bones – relaxing into the ground, and slowly breathing the spine long and the body back to its aligned state. The primary purpose, therefore, of yoga asanas is to maintain or regain health and energy, to realign posture, and to re-educate the spine and bring it back to its original suppleness. With a carefully planned practice that warms up slowly to the more difficult poses, counterbalancing backbends with forward bends, and energizing poses with quieter ones, all the systems of the body – the muscular-skeletal, cardiovascular, lymphatic, nervous, endocrine, digestive, respiratory, urinary, lymphatic, and reproductive systems – are stimulated and invigorated.

In the Taoist exercise system, complete relaxation is an absolute prerequisite for proper breath control and energy circulation, which in turn is believed to cultivate strong spiritual and mental powers. Patanjali's Yoga Sutras show how that relaxation allows you to concentrate on the infinite. Vanda Scaravelli describes a way of doing yoga poses without the slightest effort as the "song of the body." In order to sing that song, we must get quiet enough to find the rhythm of the breath and harness the exhalation to the force of gravity. Only then will we have strong enough roots to be able to lengthen, effortlessly, into each asana.

Yoga can be taken up at any age from as early as three years old to as late as seventy or eighty, and can be adapted to suit the challenges that life presents us with at each stage. The therapeutic use of yoga can have an extraordinarily positive effect on a whole range of serious illnesses and conditions, from severe asthma, high or low blood-pressure, and heart problems to cancer and multiple sclerosis, but in such cases it should be used only with the help and constant guidance of an experienced teacher and in consultation with your doctor. Much yoga practice is also invaluable during pregnancy, but again, pregnant women should always have a teacher on hand to guide them.

Essence and energy, body and breath, are indivisible: When the body does not move, essence cannot flow; when essence cannot flow, energy becomes stagnant.

SUN SSU-MO, TANG-DYNASTY PHYSICIAN

GUIDELINES FOR SAFE PRACTICE

1   *Start with simple postures and progress to the more difficult ones.*

2   *Maintain the postures as long as you can without getting tight in your body; it is only when there is a release of tension that the body moves without straining itself. Asana practice is not an endurance test. If you cannot do a pose for any length of time, release and repeat it rather than holding it in a state of tension.*

3   *Keep movements steady, slow, and deliberate. Do not lever, jerk, or bounce into a position.*

4   *Understand the purpose of each asana so that you are working with awareness and can focus on what you are doing.*

5   *Make sure that you counteract backbends with forward bends, and energizing asanas with quietening ones — you should feel neither exhausted after a practice session nor on a high.*

6   *Leave enough time at the end of your practice to quiet down in the sitting poses, with breathing and, finally, Savasana, the Corpse position.*

7   *Don't get stuck in one routine. As you progress with the yoga and it becomes a part of your life, and as the circumstances of your life change, your body will have different requirements of your daily practice.*

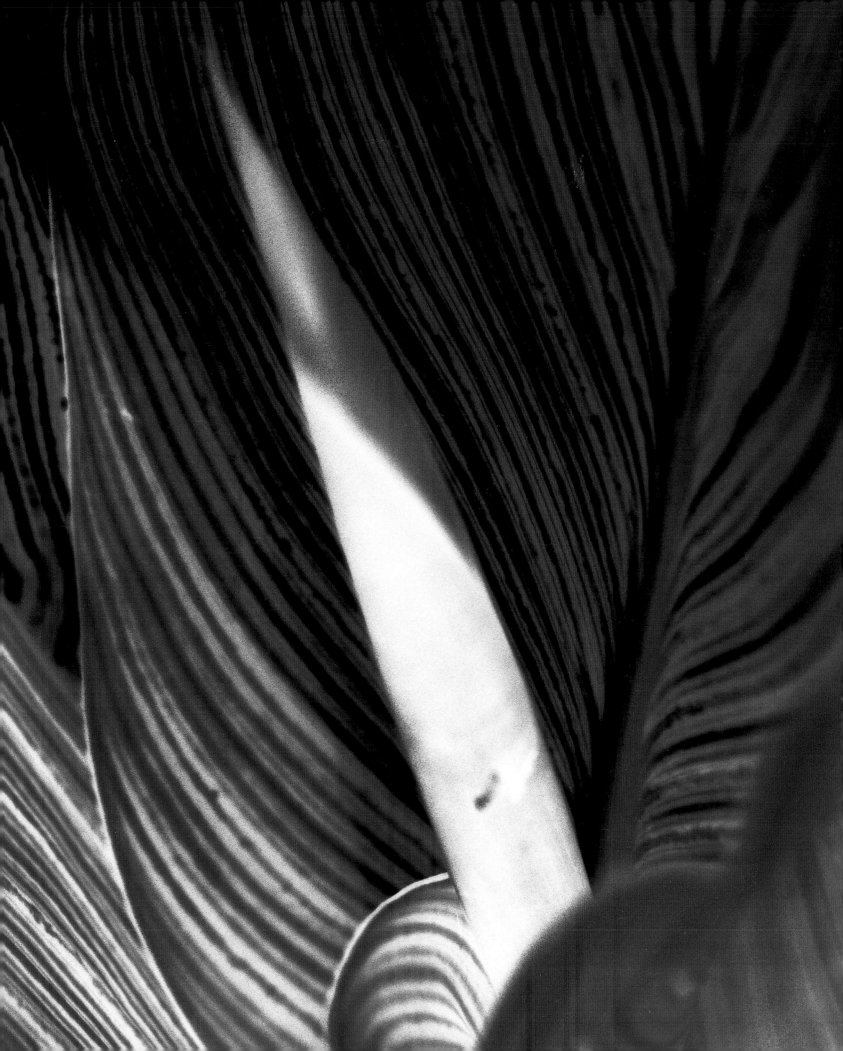

"To perform the asanas," says B.K.S. Iyengar in *Light on Yoga*, "one needs a clean, airy place, a blanket, and determination." These things really are the only prerequisites, for if you are determined, you will find the time. You need a level floor with enough space to lie full length with your arms stretched out in all directions. Wooden or warm stone floors are the best surfaces, with a blanket handy for the poses that need padding. If the floor is carpeted, or at all slippery, or if you travel a lot and never know what the next hotel bedroom floor is going to be like, you will need a non-slip mat.

You should wear loose-fitting clothes; T-shirts or tank tops, and leggings or shorts are best. Avoid wearing all-in-one outfits, because in some poses you will want to be able to feel the skin round your midriff. Always practice in bare feet. Keep socks and a blanket ready for when you get to pranayama and relaxation so that your body doesn't get chilled while you sit quietly after the hard work of the asanas. The only other prop you might want is a belt (a fabric luggage strap is perfect), and a chair to support you in poses where you are stiff.

It is better to have a regular time for practice and one that suits your schedule, so that it has a chance to become an integrated part of your daily life. Choose a time and try to stick to it. This should not be after a meal or when you are very tired. How long you practice will depend on how much time you can put aside and how experienced you are. The only rule is that it is far better to do a small amount every day, even if it is only ten minutes, than one long session every week or so. With pranayama, too, you can start with as little as five minutes a day and increase the time gradually.

THE NAMES OF THE ASANAS were not given lightly. We can learn

from them, and if we can capture the spirit of each one – Mountain, Locust, Fish, Tortoise, Lord of the Dance, or Cobra – whether it describes a living creature or a hero of Hindu mythology, we will inform our practice of the asana with it and deepen our understanding. One can go even further with the suggestion that the asana, by making us imitate the rootedness of a tree or the dance of a god, helps us to transcend our human condition. The humblest of living creatures and most common plants give their names to some of the core postures, and in the thousands of asanas that exist all creatures great and small are represented, reminding us of the awesome fact of evolution. In the philosophy of yoga, asana practice is inextricably bound up with the laws of the universe, which is why in many parts of the world it is also dedicated to the service of God.

If, as we've noted, one of the aims of asana practice is to be able to sit or stand for long periods of time, steady and serene, then the silent, still Mountain is surely the basis of all the asanas. Standing completely still and evenly on two feet which are broad and anchored securely to the ground can teach you, in the simplest and most profound way possible, to experience the three basic principles of yoga asana practice – grounding, breathing, and lengthening the spine. There is no hiding from these basics in an asana as straightforward as this one. And for this reason, many advanced practitioners of yoga find Tadasana one of the hardest.

Tada, the mountain, is the quintessence of stillness and stability. In some ancient traditions it also symbolizes the line that connects heaven and earth. Mountains are powerful and awesome because of their very silence and solidity and the way they seem to reach from the depths of the earth, right up into the heavens. Traditionally it is to the mountains of Tibet that Hindu and Buddhist sages have retreated in search of enlightenment. In the Western tradition, too, Achilles is one of several heroes of Ancient Greece thought to have been born and raised on a mountain, and think also of Moses on Mount Sinai.

So, in Mountain pose, the feet are shoulder-width apart, the toes spread wide, feet really connecting with the floor and the backs of the knees open without being locked. The body is erect but relaxed, quiet and strong. Keep your neck and shoulders soft, and as you find your center of gravity the weight of your head balances easily on your neck. With every exhalation you feel gravity pulling your feet down into the floor and drawing your tailbone downward, while above the waist you grow up toward the sky. The lengthening of the spine happens effortlessly as you breathe, helping you to find perfect stability. This natural elongation away from a solid base is what you aspire to in every asana. The first stage of all the standing poses is a few moments of quiet grounding in Tadasana.

TADASANA
Mountain

Mountains like these and travelers in the mountains and events that happen to them here are found not only in Zen literature but in the tales of every major religion. The allegory of a physical mountain for a spiritual one that stands between each soul and its goal is an easy and natural one to make.
ZEN AND THE ART OF MOTORCYCLE MAINTENANCE. ROBERT M. PIRSIG

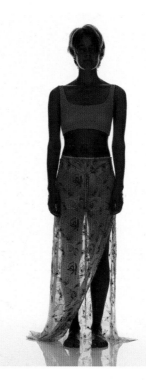

Great things are done when men and mountains meet.

WILLIAM BLAKE

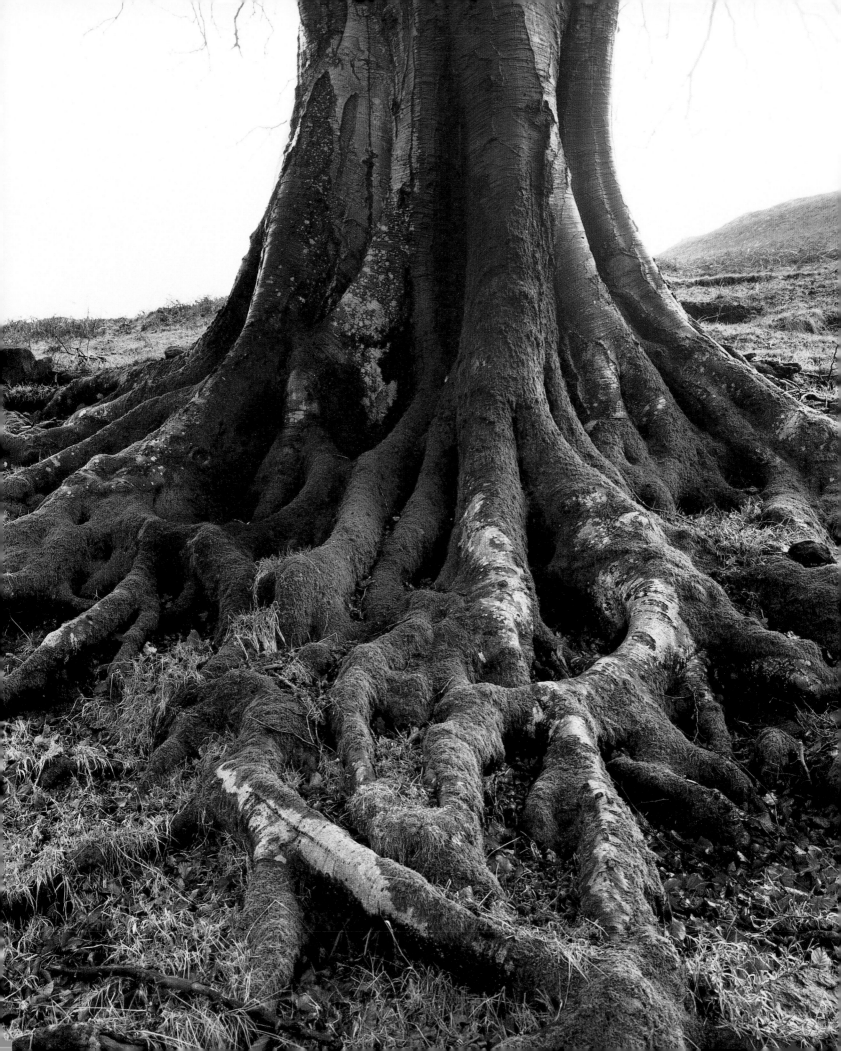

VRKSASANA
Tree

Vrksasana, as its name implies, teaches you how to ground yourself. Try to visualize the toes of your standing leg lengthening away along the ground like the roots of this extraordinary tree.

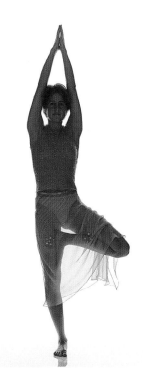

Above all things, a tree is rooted to the ground; its trunk, however tall or thin, short or broad, is utterly stable and secure. So it is with Tree pose. It is the roots, the standing foot, that allow the trunk to stay stable and the branches to grow upward toward the sky. Without roots, a tree would be carried off by the wind in its branches. And these solid foundations give trees longevity: The oak and the chestnut are capable of living for hundreds of years. A mature oak tree can weigh thirty tons, cover two thousand square yards, and comprise twenty-miles' worth of roots and branches.

To balance on one leg in this pose it is vital that the whole of the standing foot is earthed, the heels, balls of the feet, and toes all working to maintain stability, to root your foot into the ground. Gravity draws the standing leg downward, and again the spine lengthens upward from the waist. The core of the body is quiet and stable, while the groin of the bent leg stays soft and care is taken not to tip forward and stick the bottom out. By focusing quietly on a spot in the middle distance, and by breathing evenly, you find balance creeping up on you, and your arms can spread like the branches of a tree upward toward the light. As with all asymmetrical asanas, it is important to do Vrksasana on both sides so that the body develops evenly.

Trees receive their nourishment from both above and below, from sunlight and from the water in the earth.

JUDITH HARRIS

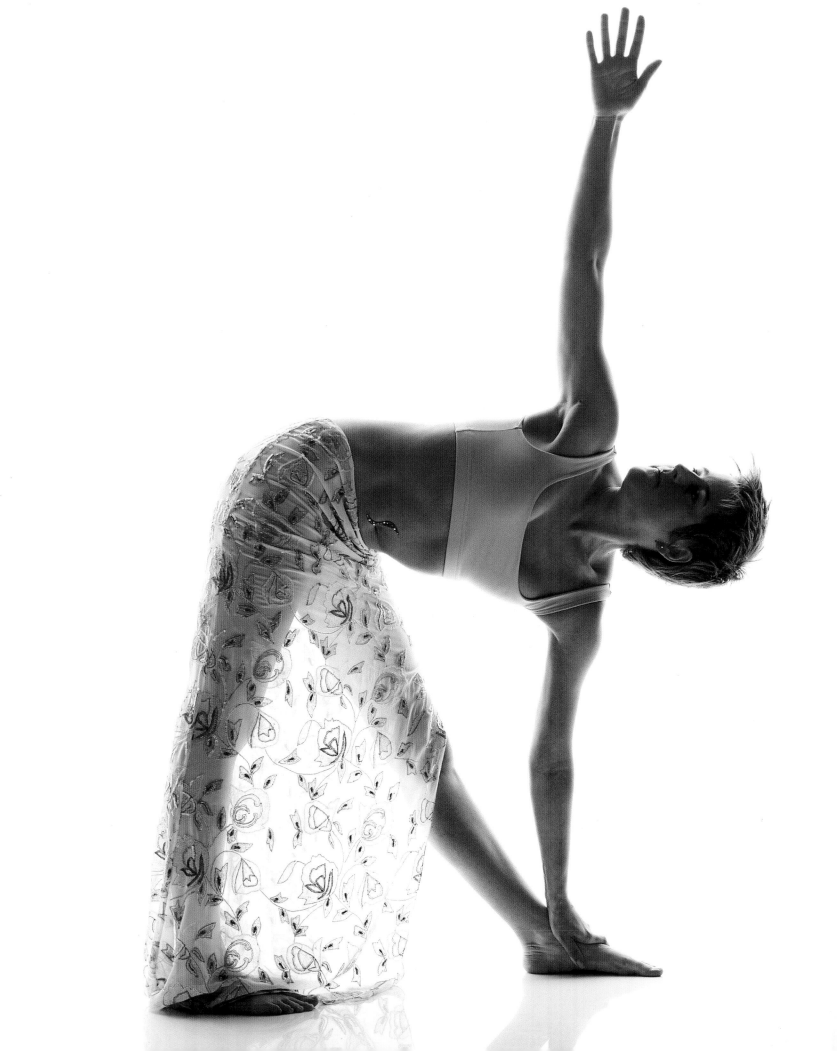

Trikonasana is one of several very strong, intense standing poses. Although these poses play a central role in many modern yoga methods, they do not appear in the earliest texts and yoga asana manuals. Some people believe that they were incorporated into the yoga system as late as the beginning of the twentieth century, inspired by the fiercer movements of martial arts exercises and the gymnastic exercises performed by the British Army in India. Nevertheless, the triangle is a significant shape in the yogic concept of the universe, representing the three tendencies of rajas, sattva, and tamas – activity, clarity, and inertia – that make up the universe. When these three qualities are in balance there is harmony. On the cosmic level, their balance – or imbalance – defines the state of the universe; on the human level it defines our individual state of mind. The Shri Yantra symbolizes this in a classic geometric form made out of layers of interconnecting triangles representing the layers of consciousness. It is used as a visual focus for the mind during meditation.

You can see how this asana got its name from the shape the body is making, leaving perfect triangles in the negative spaces between the arms and the legs. Trikonasana is one of the first of the standing poses, and is an exercise in elongating the spine by anchoring the back heel and extending away from the hips. Although the pose moves from an upright position into a sideways one, with the weight firmly on the back foot, the principle of lengthening and breathing is exactly the same as if you had remained in Tadasana; the spine stays absolutely straight, lengthening down toward the base in one direction and up to the top of the head in the other, in one long line. It is not necessary to aim for the floor in this pose; indeed, that becomes a waste of time if by doing so you bend the spine. Better to go a little way, keeping the spine straight and long at all times, feeling it move with the ebbing and flowing of the breath. This is how you will learn to unravel a tense body with simple exhalation and inhalation.

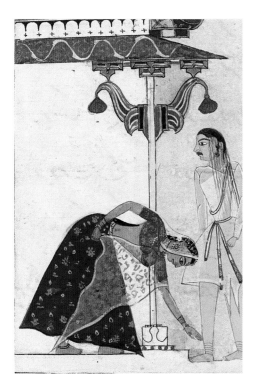

TRIKONASANA
Triangle

Although not consciously doing Trikonasana, this sixteenth-century lady bending down to touch the foot of her consort apparently knows that she must keep her heels down if she is to exert herself in this way without hurting her back.

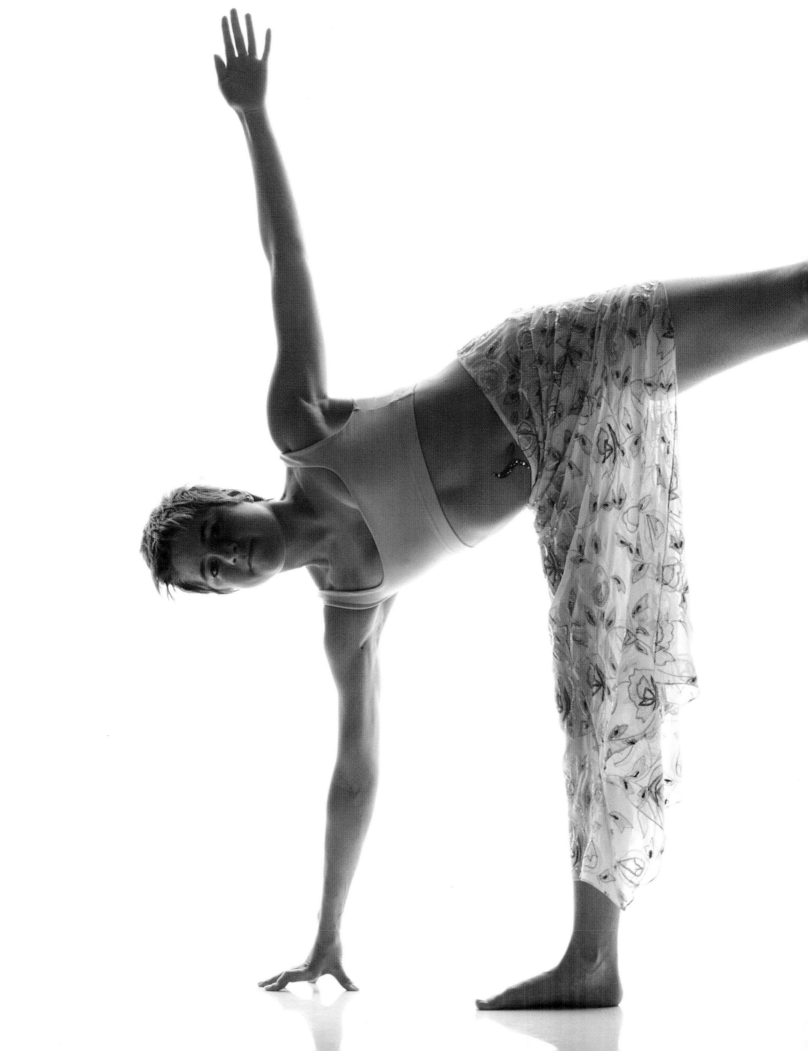

Hand in hand, on the edge of the sand,
They danced by the light of the moon,
The moon,
The moon,
They danced by the light of the moon.

THE OWL AND THE PUSSYCAT. EDWARD LEAR

Chandra is the Sanskrit for moon, and *ardha* means half. Drawing a line from the tips of the model's upper fingers to the back foot, and from there to the tips of the fingers on the floor describes the circumference of the half moon. Since there is a Sun Salutation in yoga, it is not surprising that there should also be poses devoted to the moon, a powerful symbol for the cyclical principle and the feminine aspect of nature, the life-giving and the life-taking.

Half-moon pose is a development of both Trikonasana and Virabhadrasana, Warrior pose. When doing it from Trikonasana, you place your fingers on the floor and transfer all the weight of your body on to the front leg while the back leg lengthens out behind. This releases the upper body deeper into the twist it found during Trikonasana and allows for a fantastic stretch from head to toe and through one arm to the other, releasing even further between the shoulder blades as you turn to look up at your hand. From Virabhadrasana, you take both hands lightly toward the floor, keeping your back leg long and strong – think of it as your rudder! Then you turn to face forward, opening the upper arm up to the sky.

ARDHA CHANDRASANA
Half Moon

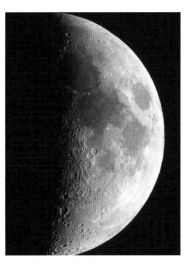

The curvaceous softness of this half moon is echoed in the sensuous silhouette of the female form.

To bend your spine so far back that you meet the floor behind you without relinquishing the ground under your heels is a movement that takes the standing poses to their ultimate conclusion; the heels root so deeply that when you have grown upward as far as your height allows, there is only one way to continue to find length, and that is by pouring the body into a slow, effortless backbend. Vanda Scaravelli was at one time a pupil of B.K.S. Iyengar and later went on to develop her own method of yoga with great emphasis on gravity and the breath. Legend has it that Iyengar described hers as "the best body for yoga that I have ever seen," and the fluidity with which she does the poses, even though here she is in her eighties, is inspiring, to say the least. She describes the movement of going into a backbend from Tadasana as a "wave" of the body. In her inspirational book *Awakening the Spine*, she gives these instructions:

It is about the way the spine moves from the heels to the top of the head with gravity. You let the body sink, sink, sink. The upper part becomes lighter the more you sink. As the upper part of the body becomes light there is a beautiful wave in the body, and the body moves with the wave. The wave to the ground allows gravity into and through the spine. All the energy goes to the head. The body is pulled down to the ground and from the waist up there is a most wonderful feeling, of behaving and of moving. This feeling gives a sense of authority, of freedom, and of beauty. The more we are able to breathe down into the heels the more the upper body will be free to stretch and release upward.

By practicing the pose in this way, and by visualizing the dramatic pull of the water on ocean waves as they curve up, up away from the surface of the sea and then over before they drop down again, you will discover that there is no exhaustion from the effort or pinching in the back. Rather, there is an extraordinary feeling of lightness and renewed energy.

URDHVA DHANURASANA
Backbend from Standing

*movements are like waves
you have to go with them*

SANDRA SABATINI

*It is hard to believe
that Vanda Scaravelli
is in her eighties as
she demonstrates
Urdhva Dhanurasana
from standing
with awesome power
and energy.*

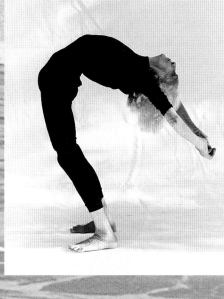

FEET ~ Our feet are intricate structures of fifty-two small bones each bound by four layers of muscle. The mechanism is a miracle combination of strength and flexibility, designed to support the weight of the whole body, to maintain its balance, to propel it in motion, and to act as shock absorbers. To do their job efficiently the feet must be alive, supple, and springy; otherwise, their weakness will transmit up through the legs and into the hips and the rest of the body, throwing the whole structure out of alignment. Through the practice of yoga the feet gradually begin to come alive; the toes regain the independence of movement that they were born with, the arches lift, the ankles strengthen. It is also mostly through our feet that we feel the ground, our ultimate support. To be stable and solid on our feet is to feel secure and confident at a very fundamental and profound level, giving us the base from which to walk tall through life. To achieve the sort of movement described on the previous page is inconceivable unless you have learned to establish a powerful connection between your feet and the floor.

Why, then, do most of us neglect them? Anyone who has suffered so much as an ingrown toenail knows how we take our feet for granted most of the time, and how incapacitated we are when they cause us problems. Given their elemental importance, you would think that a large, wide, muscle-bound foot would be the ultimate aesthetic, and yet the foot has been the subject of fetishism and distortion; the idealized foot is small, delicate, and soft, not a functioning clod-hopper. The most famously extreme example of this comes from China, where it was the custom to bind women's feet from early childhood so that they remained tiny and became squashed-up to the point of deformity, thereby incapacitating the women. Throughout history, small, soft feet have been the erotic ideal, representing class, a life of leisure, and beauty. "I don't love you coz your feet's too big," goes the jazz song. Until recently in the Western world – where most people can afford shoes – women particularly have stuffed their feet into shoes that are too small, squashed their toes into sharp points, and thrown the balance of their whole weight onto towering heels with tiny stiletto bases, forcing them to walk with their bottoms stuck out and their hips swaying. Not only does this put intolerable strain on their lower backs and knees, but it clearly restricts freedom of movement both practically and symbolically. Anthropologists may be excused for equating these dictates of Western fashion with the indignities once inflicted on women in China.

But there are many places in the world still, especially in cultures where it is normal to walk barefoot, as in India, in which beautiful feet are portrayed as strong, sinuous, and flexible. This is particularly true of representations of the Buddha, as if real enlightenment were only possible with lovely wide, grounded feet.

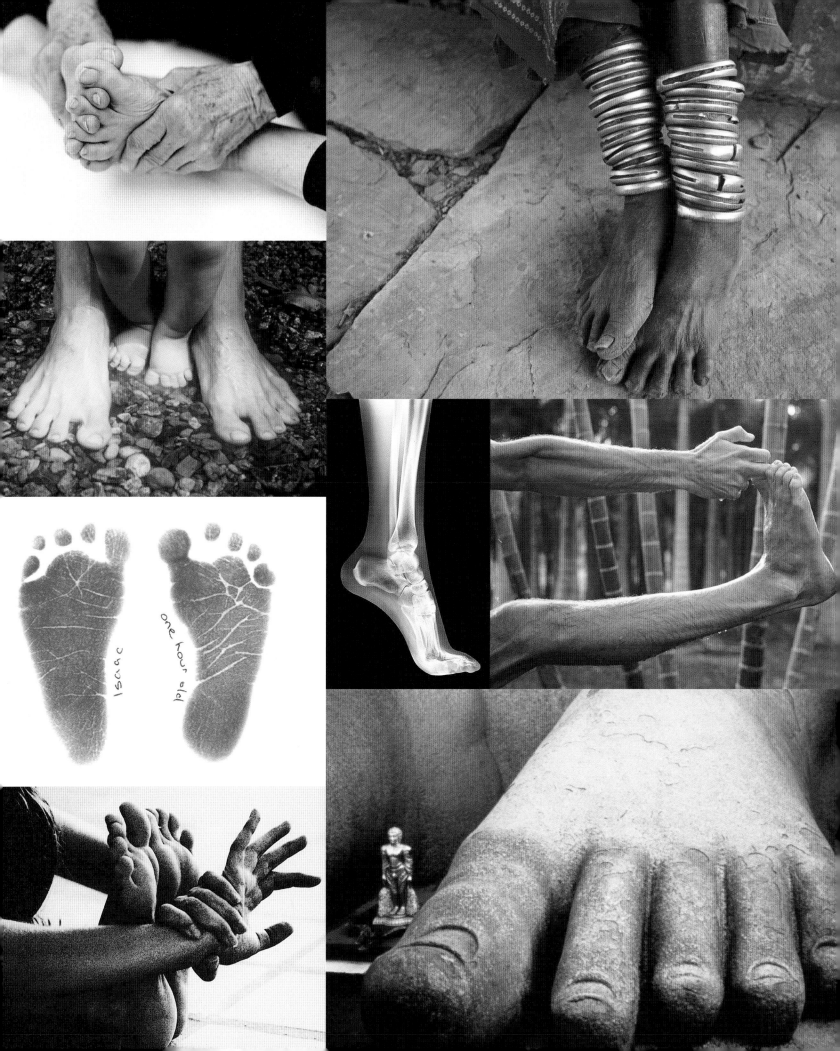

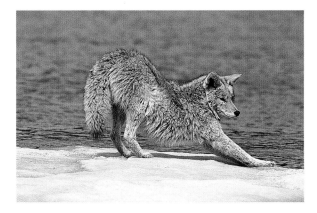
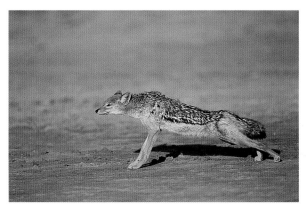

Just watch a dog getting up after it has been sleeping and give itself a stretch. It puts its front paws out in front, sticks its bottom in the air, and lets its back stretch all the way along the space in between. In other words, it looks pretty much like Svanasana. The movement is instinctive and fluid. Look at the dog's silhouette. As long as it is still stretching and hasn't relaxed into inviting a game, it never sticks out its chest in an attempt to touch the floor. Some people do the asana this way, thinking it is impressive to be able reach the floor with the chest. However, this is not the point of Svanasana, for unless you are extraordinarily bendy, it will only shorten the lengthening that can take place at the back of the body. The feet and palms of the hands should be wide and flat on the floor and the backs of the knees open to anchor the hips. The front ribs stay soft and the shoulders must be relaxed and free. Dog pose gives you energy. It is a lovely asana for really feeling the stretch from the tailbone to the top of the neck in one line as you exhale and reach further and further. It is also a very good asana to warm-up with before doing the inverted poses.

Often a dog will do a sequence of stretches when it gets up, first with its head down as described, and then bringing its weight forward over its front paws, stretching out its lower back and hind legs. This is such an intense and long stretch of the spine that it turns into a mini backbend, as the jackal above so effortlessly shows. It is important to breathe out as you go into this pose, drawing your abdomen in to relieve the pressure caused by overbending in your lumbar spine. Dog is, of course, one of the integral poses in the cycle of the sun salutation. Though at once dynamic and energizing, it is also very beneficial for relieving tension in the neck because of the way the head can hang freely and the throat and face relax as the chest opens and the shoulders release. For this reason it is a good pose to do after Headstand or when the neck is feeling stiff. In many more-athletic yoga classes, Adho Mukha Svanasana is used as a preparation for jumping into Chataranga Dandasana; but it is a shame not to enjoy it for its own sake, as an exceptional stretch that tones the legs and back of ankles, opens the chest, massages the abdominal muscles, and increases circulation to the head and face.

The familiar morning stretch common to all dogs combines an effortless grace with a luxurious elongation of the spine.

ADHO MUKHA SVANASANA

Dog

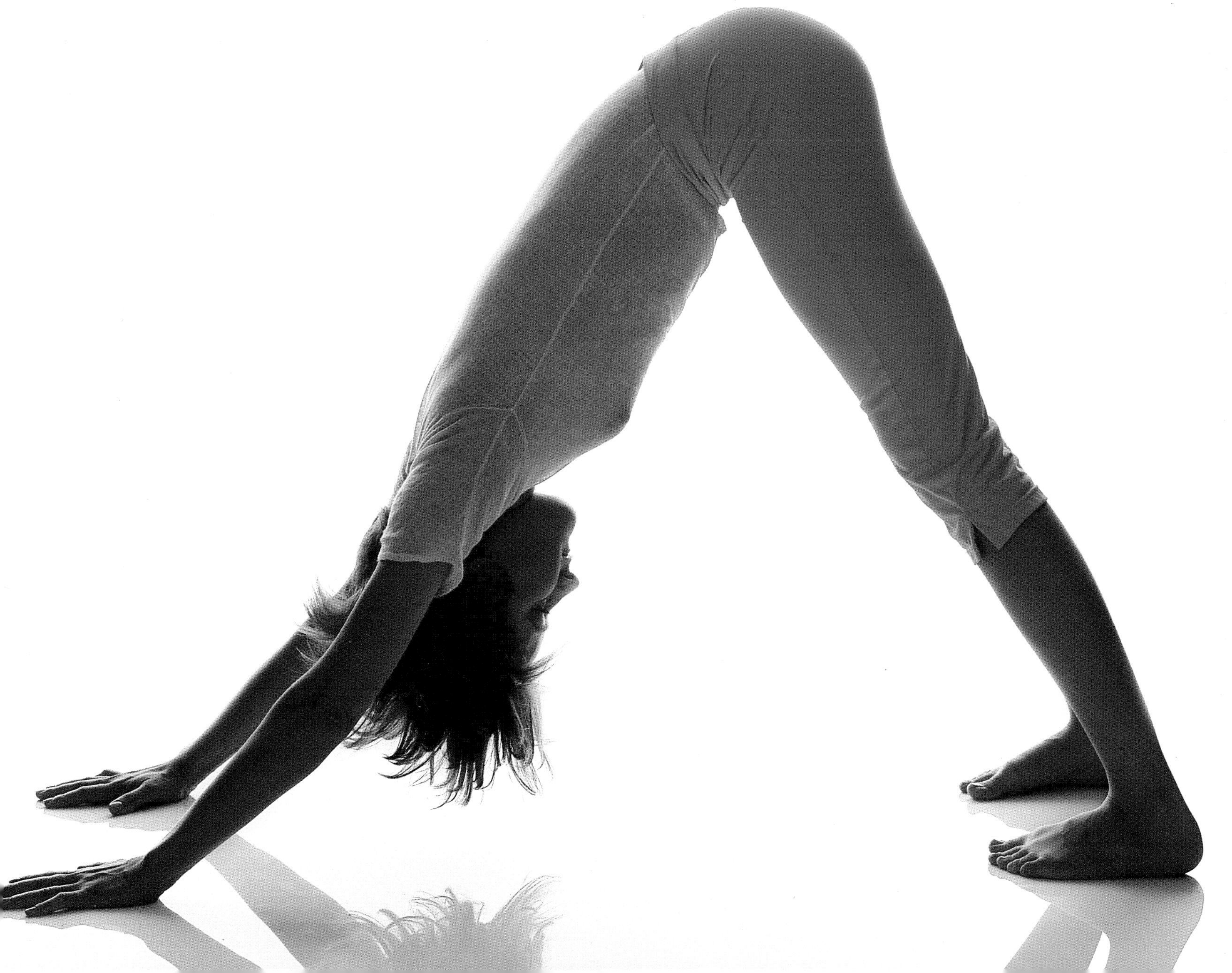

Salamba Sarvangasana was known by the sages as the mother or queen of the asanas. They believed it developed the female qualities of patience and emotional stability, and strove for harmony in the body the way a mother strives for harmony in the family. A rejuvenating pose, it massages the thyroid glands and restores balance, especially if you practice it enough so that you can stay in it for some time. After a long and stressful day, a ten-minute Shoulderstand can be a powerful restorative provided you go into it without tensing your neck and shoulders. Salamba Sarvangasana is a counterpose for Headstand and should always be practiced after Headstand, but it is also one of the asanas that a beginner can work on long before Headstand has been mastered.

It is important that the body is lying straight on the floor before you go into Salamba Sarvangasana, and that the neck and shoulders are not tense or compressed. Let your arms and shoulders lengthen away from your neck. The more time you spend lying breathing and lengthening before you roll your feet over your head and come up the better, and never turn or adjust your head while up there.

Once you have taken your legs up, your elbows become your roots. It is by giving your elbows and shoulders away to the floor that you will feel gravity anchoring you; the more you exhale into your elbows, the farther you will be able to walk your palms up your back and the higher you will get with the front of your thighs. This must of course be done without putting pressure on your neck or tensing the jaw. Once you are comfortable and upright enough to be able to relax a little in the pose, try to feel that the place where the palms of your hands come into contact with your back is a meeting point between two quiet surfaces, rather than that the back is collapsing into the hands or the hands are digging and shoving into the back.

SALAMBA SARVANGASANA
Shoulderstand

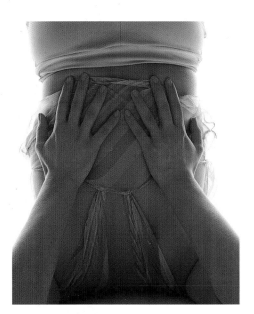

At the still point of the turning world.
   Neither flesh nor fleshless;
Neither from nor towards; at the still point,
   there the dance is,
But neither arrest nor movement.

"BURNT NORTON," T.S. ELIOT

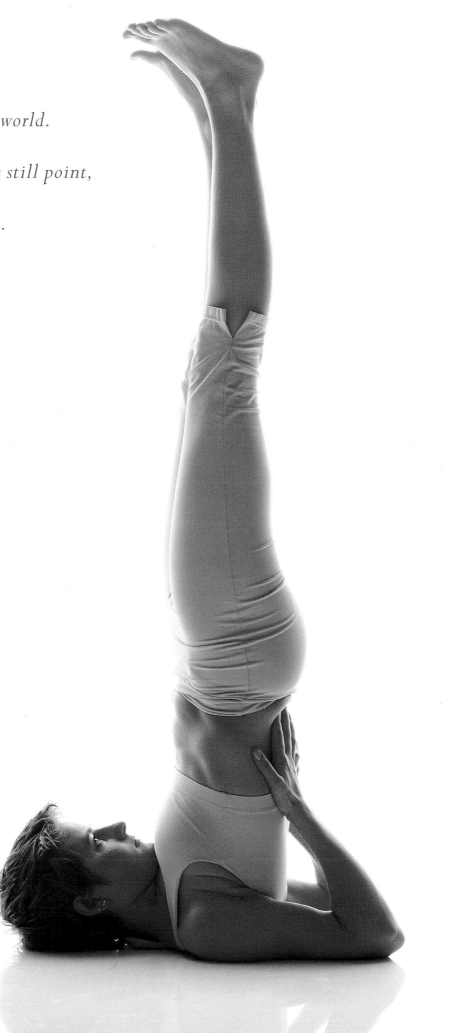

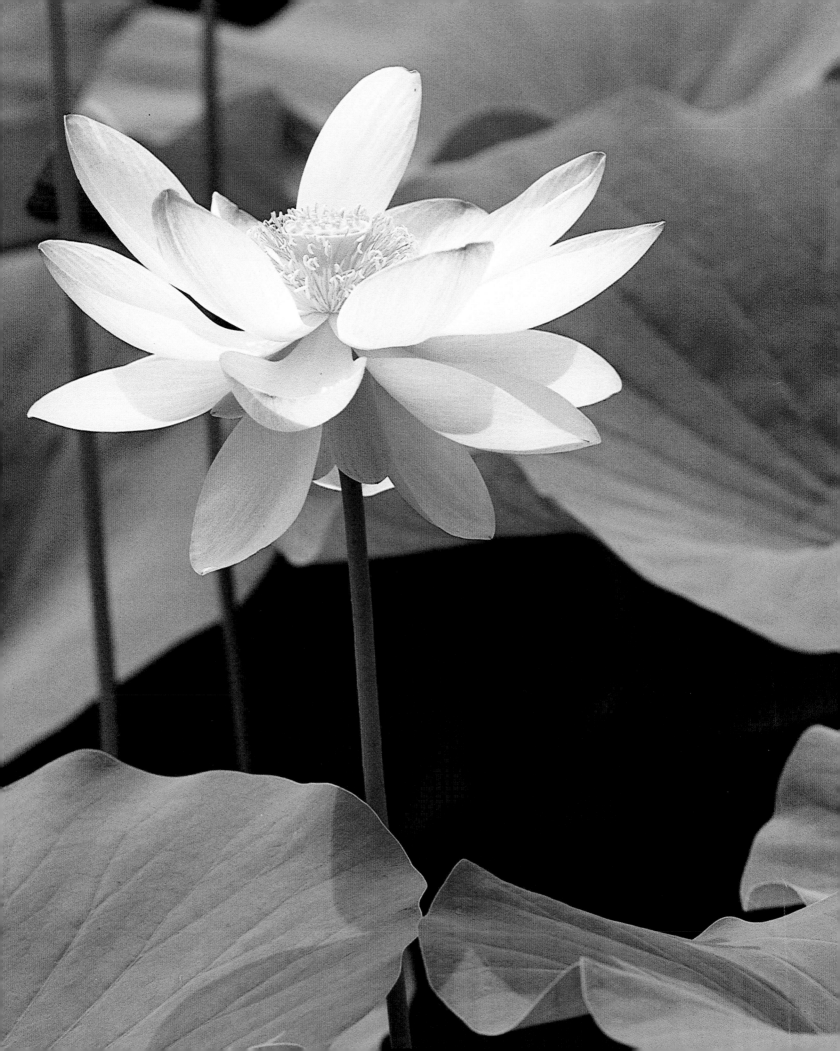

*Worked using gravity
and energy, the body
can open up like
the petals of a lotus
blossom on a seemingly
fragile stem.*

URDHVA PADMASANA IN SARVANGASANA
Lotus Backbend in Shoulderstand

When you can do Salamba Sarvangasana easily, you
will be able to get further freedom and strength
from its variations. Lotus Backbend is one of a range
of variations that can be done in Shoulderstand.
When properly carried out, it gets to a point in
the back of the spine between the shoulderblades
that is difficult to lengthen in other poses.

The diagonal backbend in Shoulderstand can
be done either with the legs stretched out
straight, or in Padmasana, as illustrated. With the
sacrum resting in one hand, the hips can open at
the front so that the legs travel away from the
core of the body, and whole spine elongates. As in
simple Shoulderstand, it is important not to let
the shoulders and neck get tight. This asana must
be done in both directions and with the lotus legs
crossed both ways.

When you start practicing yoga is it difficult
to stay in even a simple Shoulderstand for any
length of time, both because of lack of stamina
and because it takes time to learn how to breathe
evenly in the postures. After a while, the asanas
become more fluid and make more sense. You
learn to combine the actions of the body and the
ebbing and flowing of the breath in one movement,
and it begins to look and feel easy. Then the
whole sequence of Shoulderstand variations can be
done as one continuous action.

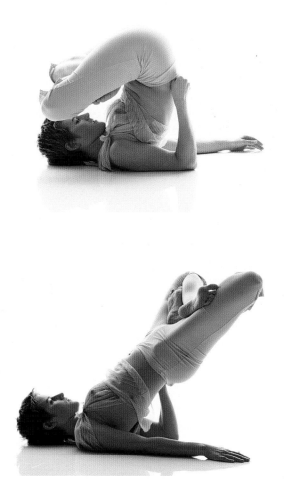

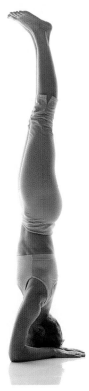

If Shoulderstand is the queen of the asanas, then Headstand is the king, and the most important of the inverted poses. Most simply put, Headstand is Tadasana upside down, and should feel as straight, stable, and strong as Tadasana, with all the focus at the back of the body, the chest and abdomen remaining quiet and soft. It should produce a feeling of lightness and freedom, but it can be quite stimulating, which is why it is always followed by the more relaxing Shoulderstand.

I have been to classes where Shoulderstand is not taught after Headstand and there is no doubt that this results in an imbalance. Each pose has its counterpose, which stretches the body in the opposite way or calms an energizing movement. Headstand without Shoulderstand can leave you buzzing and over-aggressive.

As with Shoulderstand, it is vital that you go into Headstand slowly, establishing a solid base before you lift. The forearms are placed on the floor with the elbows no further than shoulder-width apart and the fingers interlaced, leaving the wrists in contact with the floor. The secure base that this provides allows for the neck and shoulders to release, the arms to lengthen away from the shoulders, and the weight to drop more into the elbows with every exhalation. The elbows are the roots of this pose, and the more weight that goes into them, the more the neck is freed and the head relieved of pressure at the base of the straightening and stretching spine.

Headstand also shares with Shoulderstand its capacity for a large number of variations: leg-stretches, twists, and backbends, many of which can be done in Lotus as well as with straight legs. All of these are particularly helpful for those with knee or hip problems, because they allow for these joints to be worked without any weight on them.

SIRSASANA
Headstand

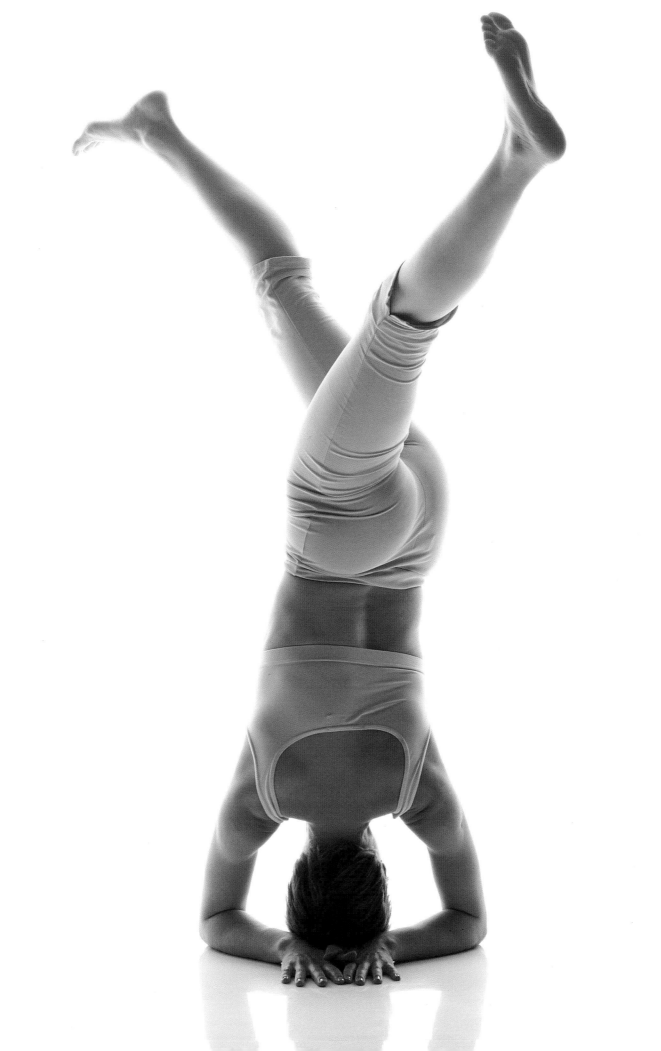

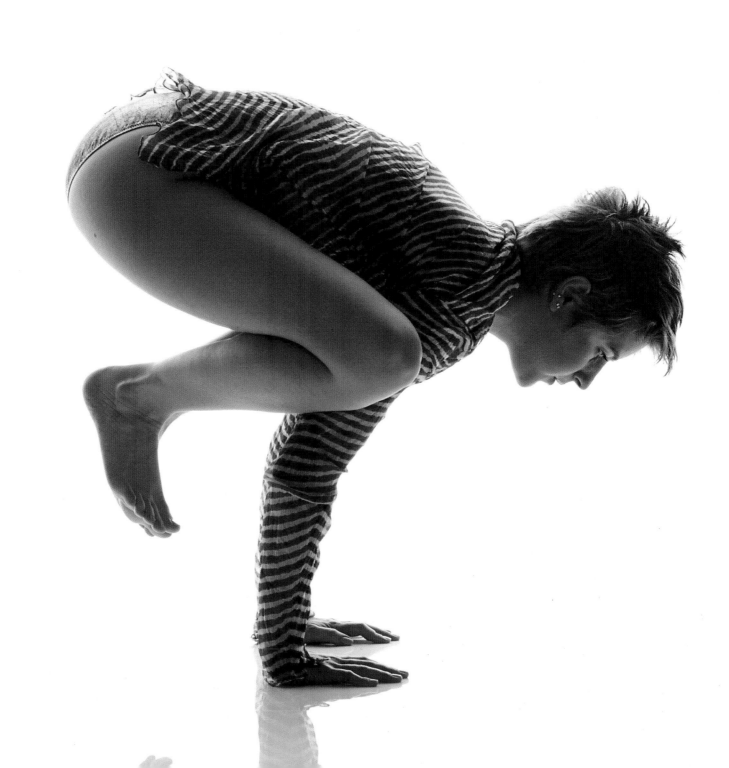

Many yoga poses are inspired by the natural movements of animals, as if the sages, by naming them this way, were encouraging practitioners of yoga to return to an instinctive sense of how the body moves, from the inside out. In Bakasana, the base of the pose is in the hands, fingers spread out like the crane's claws, and long, leglike arms. As the heels of the hands give themselves to the ground and the arms straighten, the spine rounds into the body of the bird, with the tailbone drawing down toward the floor. The balance comes with a powerful exhalation, as the abdomen is pulled in and the knees grip the arms. While you work on this asana, see the bird in your mind's eye with its long legs and extended nape of the neck. This crowned crane is graceful and majestic.

Many yoga asanas can be arranged in a sequence. Some of these start out with simpler poses, which prepare for the technically more difficult ones that come later. Although it is not important to do the more advanced poses, it is interesting to see how a sequence develops. Bakasana is part of a cycle that starts in Tadasana, from where the knees bend and the bottom drops all the way down into a squat. In squat, the hands are placed flat on the floor with the fingers spread, and the knees grip the outsides of the upper arms so that the weight of the body

can be transferred from the feet onto the hands and the arms lengthened into Crane. While still in Crane, the crown of the head is placed on the floor beyond the hands, and the weight is distributed between the hands and the head so that the legs lengthen up to form a three-point Headstand. Finally, to complete the cycle, the legs come over the head and onto the floor on the other side to make the Headstand Backarch, from where the strongest and most supple people root the heels and, with a powerful exhalation, come back up to Tadasana. This last stage of the cycle is one that only people who have practiced regularly for many years can hope to achieve.

Just when you feel you've mastered one yoga asana, you realize that there is another level to work on and learn from. Once you can do Bakasana from Headstand, try Urdhva Kukkutasana, in which the legs are put into Lotus before the body curls down for the thighs to rest on the tops of the arms as they did in Bakasana. This pose is named after the strutting cock.

BAKASANA
Crane

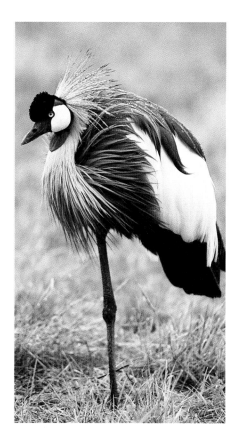

Left. This illustrates with extraordinary clarity how the hands have become the feet of the pose.

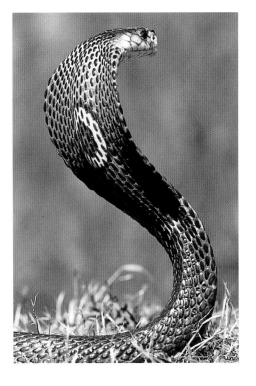

Feel the sheer weight of body this spectacled cobra leaves on the ground as it rears up to strike its prey.

Once again, the secret of this pose lies in its name. You need only imagine the rippling movement a snake makes as it slithers along to understand the reptilian movement with which this pose is concerned. In preparation for Bhujangasana you lie face-down on the floor, feeling exactly this rippling of the spine as the inhalation and exhalation move up and down the back of the body. When the cobra strikes, it is the weight of its coiled body on the ground that gives it the strength to rear up the rest of its great length and open its hood over its prey. Like the cobra, you must keep your lower body heavy, motionless, and strong as you move in to strike. You breathe out, giving your hands away to the floor and lengthening the head, neck, and upper back upward as you do so, allowing the chest to open and leaving the heavy base behind on the floor. As the spine lengthens, the tailbone presses down, and the upper back feels wonderfully free. The movement is slow and sinuous, the spine moving as one coordinated whole. If any pinching is felt at the back of the waist it is a sign that you are pushing into the pose and damaging your lumbar vertebrae.

Salabhasana, the Locust pose, is the precursor to Cobra and is the backbend with the subtlest body movement, arms and upper body lifted slightly off the floor. Do it with the legs left behind as with Cobra, or with the legs lifting and lengthening away from the back of the waist. When done properly, this is a very intense stretch in both directions.

… earth brown, earth-golden from the burning bowels of the earth…
[He] looked around like a god, unseeing, into the air,
*   And slowly turned his head,*
And slowly, very slowly, as if thrice adream,
*   Proceeded to draw his slow length curving round*
And climb again the broken bank of my wall-face…
*   snake-easing his shoulders*

"SNAKE," D.H. LAWRENCE

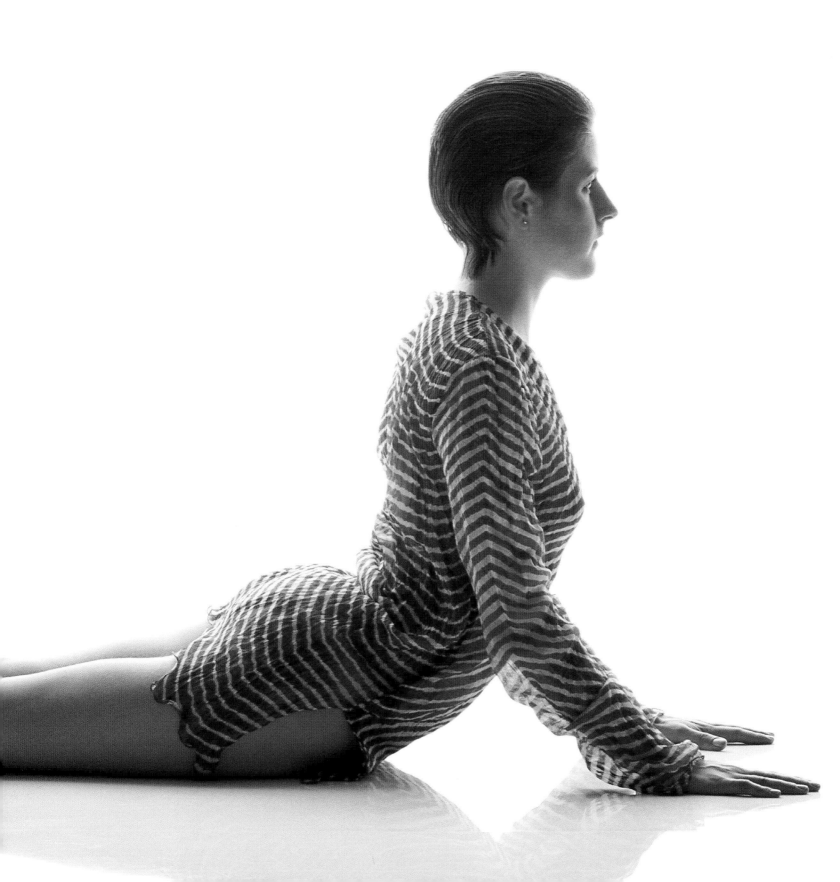

Ancient civilizations as far apart as Pharaonic Egypt and Viking Europe celebrated this invigorating movement in their art, showing, once again, that yoga did not have a monopoly on such movements but only enlarged upon man's natural inclination to work the body in poses that would calm or stimulate.

Just as a bow arcs from the pull of the bowstring on each end of it, in Urdhva Dhanurasana the back bends because gravity acts like a bowstring on the hands and feet, plugging them into the floor, drawing them down and making it inevitable that the spine lengthen upward into an arch. Once one has learned to do this pose in tune with the breath, going up into this pose, with one smooth exhalation, is as effortless as the flight of an arrow from the thrust of the bow string, and the body looks strong and free. The whole movement is fluid and graceful, one that harnesses the power of gravity rather than pushing and straining against it.

Many people do this pose with the heels coming up off the floor, the feet turning out and the lower spine pinching. The feet must remain glued to the ground and parallel with each other, and the knees mustn't fall outward; the body must go up into a smooth arch in which the chest and hips are level and there is an even extension of the spine with no pushing into the lower back.

We all spend far too much time hunched over and bending forward. The fronts of our bodies are constantly receiving stimulation, and it is from here that most of us initiate our movements and orientate ourselves. Jung made a connection between this and the distant relationship most of us have with our unconscious when he wrote, "'Behind' is the region of the unseen, the unconscious." To open out the back is enormously energizing and recharging, so much so that if you don't counterbalance the backbends with forward bends, you may find it difficult to calm down.

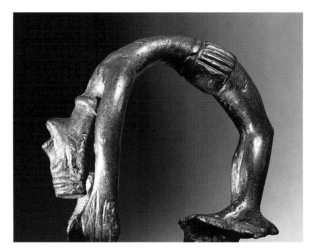

All the freedom and joy of Urdhva Dhanurasana is evident in this Viking bronze sculpture of the movement.

URDHVA DHANURASANA
Bow

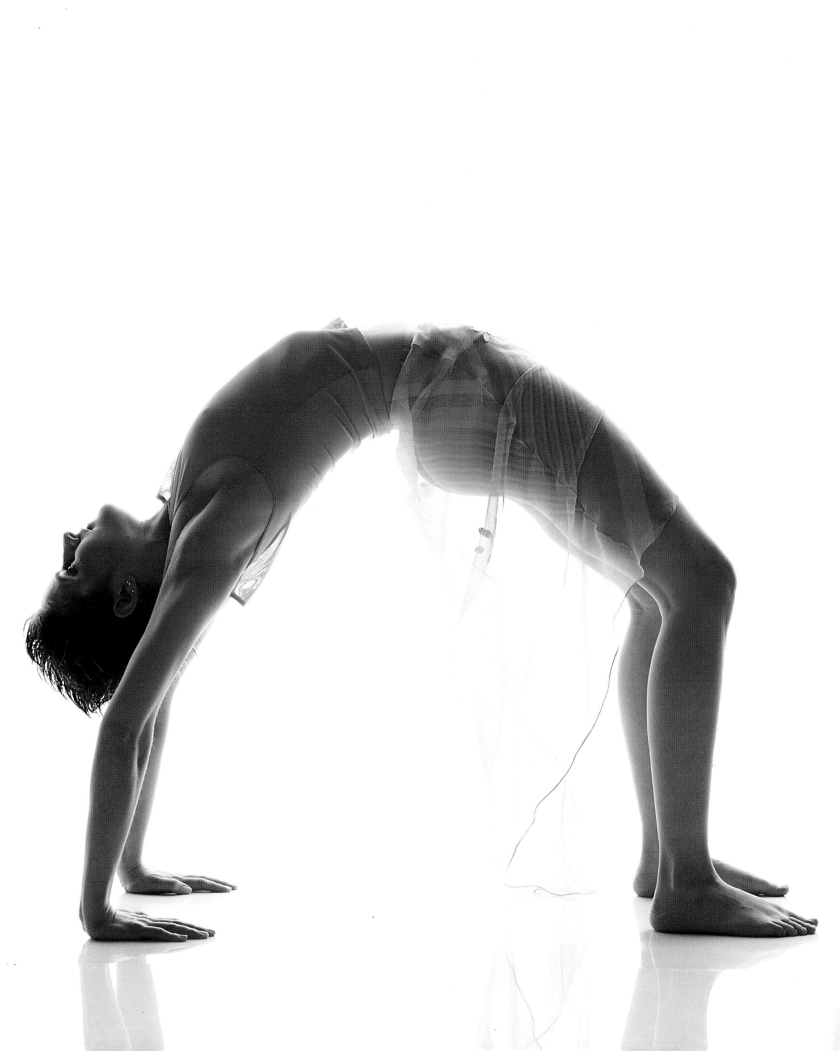

A *kapota* is a dove or pigeon, so Rajakapotasana is the king of the pigeons, and *eka pada* means "one leg" or "one foot." This asana is as demanding as it is beautiful, requiring an intense elongation of the spine into a backbend that opens the chest out, wholly capturing the spirit of the strutting pigeon. The final stage of Eka Pada Rajakapotasana is arrived at through a sequence of three stages, in which the backbend gets progressively more intense. It is essential that one feel really secure and free in each stage before moving on to the one that follows. As the Persian mystic Rumi explained so eloquently, it is not through extra power that one will achieve, but by finding balance and harmony in the body as it is.

Take time in the first stage, with the front leg bent on the floor in front of you and the opposite leg stretched out behind, to feel your back leg lengthen away. Be sure, too, that the hips are parallel and that the back hip doesn't twist open as you take its leg back. In the second stage of the asana, when you bring your torso more upright, your center of gravity is thrown right back into your tailbone. That is where your roots are in Eka Pada Rajakapotasana, and your tailbone must move powerfully toward the floor as you breathe out, holding the pelvis heavy, in order to keep enough length in the spine for it to bend without any pinching. The movement of bending the back leg in the third stage should intensify this rooting of the base rather than cause compression in the lower back. Only once you are fully rooted in this stage of the pose do you make another powerful exhalation, lengthen your arms from the armpits, and reach them back to hold the back foot. This last movement builds on the grounding obtained by the first three stages to leave the upper spine utterly free to elongate. Being asymmetrical, this pose must be practiced on both sides.

Strong backward stretches of the lumbar and dorsal spine are very exhilarating. Physically the thyroids, parathyroids, adrenals, and gonads are all stimulated, and the muscles of the neck and shoulder are exercised. Eka Pada Rajakapotasana should be practiced toward the peak of a long yoga session, where your body is well warmed up but not yet tired. It must always be followed soon afterward by a long, quiet, forward bend, such as Paschimottanasana.

EKA PADA RAJAKAPOTASANA
Pigeon

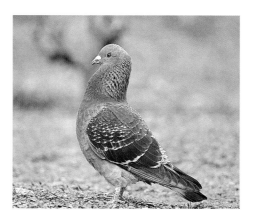

The proud stance of this ordinary pigeon suggests he sees himself as a king — a feeling wholly captured in the pose.

Tie two birds together.
They will not be able to fly,
even though they now have four wings.
JALALUDIN RUMI

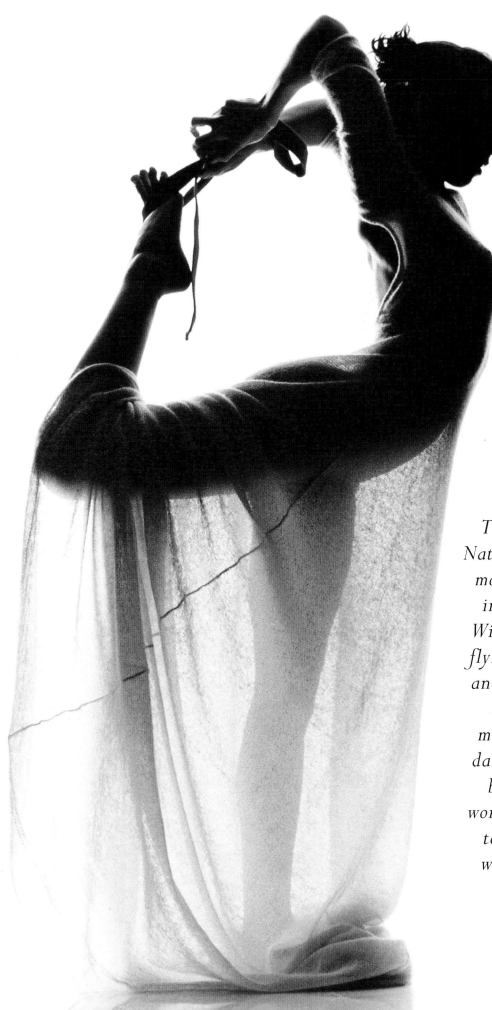

The image of Shiva
Nataraja is perhaps the
most dramatic single
image in all art…
With his matted locks
flying about furiously
and his arms and legs
in fast rhythmic
motion, Shiva is not
dancing to entertain,
but to involve the
world in his dance and
to awaken it to the
wonder of creation.

BALRAJ KHANNA

NATARAJASANA
Lord of the Dance

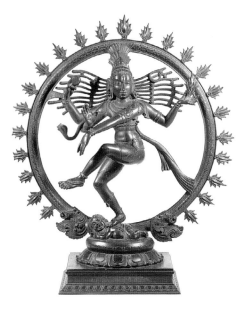

Nataraja, the Lord of the Dance, is one of the forms in which Shiva is worshipped. For Shiva is not only the Destroyer but also the Creator. All the forces of nature are concentrated within him – he is the lord of the blissful dance of the universe. In the sculpture, the Universe is symbolized by the circle of flames around the dancing figure, the dwarf under his feet represents Ignorance, and the drum in his upper right hand Time, to whose beat Shiva is dancing in his endless cycle of destruction and creation.

All of the vitality, drama, and beauty of this sculpture is present in the asana, which incorporates the strength of Warrior pose with the grace of the dance. Natarajasana is very similar to Eka Pada Rajakapotasana in its action on the body, although for most people it is easier to achieve. It is essential when doing Natarajasana not to bend at the waist but to create space there by lengthening the back thigh away from its root in the groin and finding stability and strength in the standing leg. As in Pigeon pose, the two hip bones must remain parallel. In the advanced position of this pose, the foot is held in both hands and brought to rest on the top of the head.

ARDHA MATSYENDRASANA
Sitting Twist

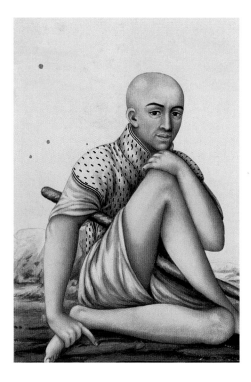

This European-style watercolor was probably painted in Lucknow in the 1790s. It shows a young gentleman practicing one of the more intense poses in which the spine twists in a movement coming from the core of the body.

The European-style seventeenth-century Indian watercolor shows how the practice of yoga asanas was integrated into Indian everyday life, and by no means reserved for the ascetics who wandered the continent in search of enlightenment. For this young gentleman to have been painted practicing it, the twist must have been considered one of the classics of the yoga asanas.

Legend has it that Shiva was on a remote island telling his consort, Parvati, about the mysteries of yoga when he noticed a fish listening motionless to what he was saying. When Shiva saw how quiet the fish was, he realized that it had learned yoga from him, and he sprinkled water on the fish, whereupon it rose up in the divine form of Matsyendra, Lord of the Fishes. From that day on, Matsyendra traveled the continent spreading knowledge of yoga, and this asana is named after him.

The key to all of the sitting twists is to feel both sitting bones making contact with the floor, and to leave the hips behind as you breathe out, draw the belly to the back of the waist, and turn with the whole spine. In her book *Yoga and You*, Esther Myers describes this movement with a very helpful image: "It is like taking the cork out of a bottle, creating space and openness as you turn."

It is essential that you don't give in to the temptation of using the bent leg as a sort of lever against which to push your arm and force the spine into a twist. Doing them in this way will sooner or later result in damage to the spine.

The therapeutic effects of the poses have been passed down by teachers for centuries, and twists like this one are particularly healing as they gently massage the liver and kidneys while also ensuring against backache, particularly lumbago, and pain in the hips. However, they should not be done during pregnancy.

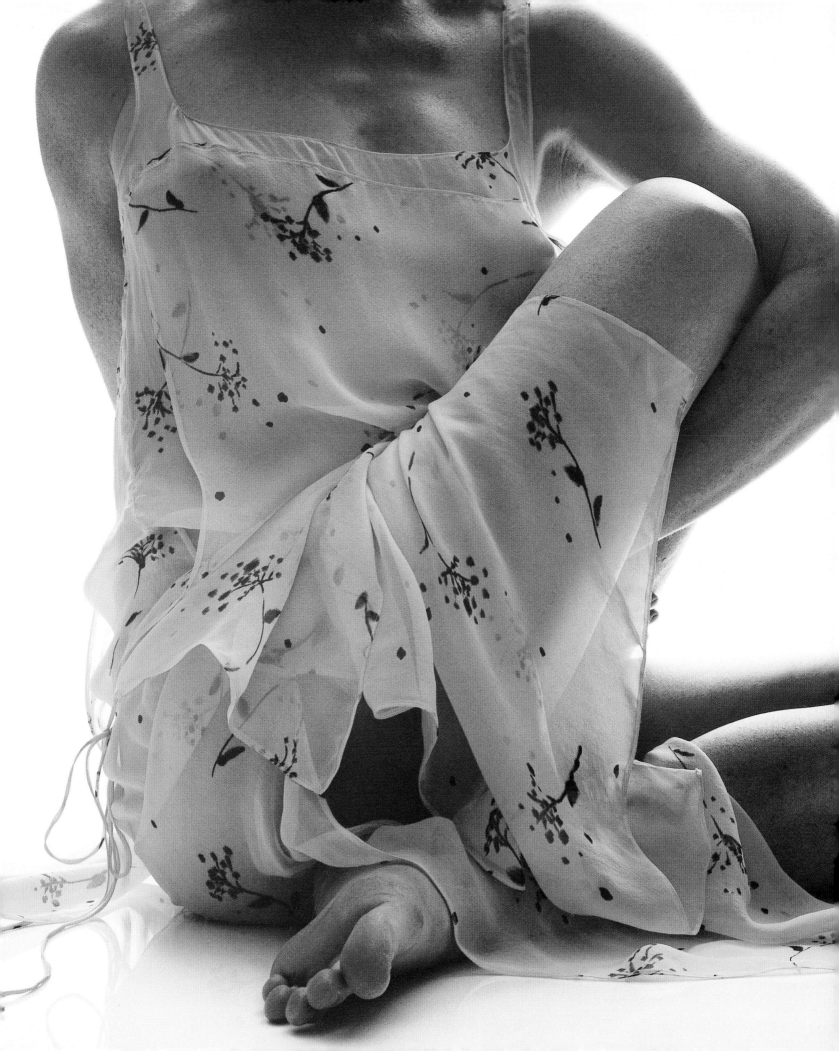

This seated Forward Bend translates as "the stretching of the west" because in India it is traditional to face east, the land of the rising sun, both to pray and to practice asanas. So the west is the whole of the back of the body, from the heels and the Achilles tendons to the crown of the head and the backs of the hands and tips of the fingers. The real purpose of this asana is to facilitate the movement of the breath in the back.

In Paschimottanasana, the two sitting bones – the hard knobs you can feel under the buttocks – become your roots. Tight hamstrings, which many Westerners, particularly male, can suffer from, make all the sitting poses that have the legs straight out along the floor extremely difficult, and

Paschimottanasana is the purest of these, providing no extra frills to distract the mind from the matter in hand. With tight hamstrings it is quite impossible to bring the torso forward without bending the knees right up off the floor. This is when people make the mistake of trying to yank themselves into the Forward Bend, striving to get their heads onto their knees by force. But this is not what the pose is about. The old adage that for yoga one must have infinite patience and no ambition is the absolute prerequisite for progress in Paschimottanasana if your hamstrings are tight. First, when you are sitting with your legs stretched straight out in front of you, the weight of the hips must anchor you down. If all you achieve at this stage is a slumped

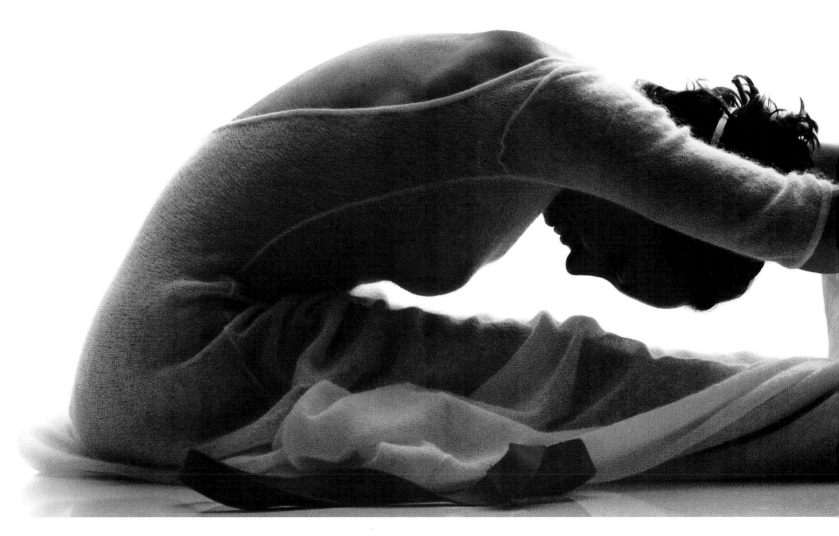

back, then lean back onto your hands and feel how the hips can weigh you down when the muscles in your back are not struggling against the hamstrings to hold you up. When you can sit upright without discomfort, feeling heavy in the base of the pose, then on the exhalation, with relaxed shoulders and a flat back, you can begin to lengthen forward, leaving the hips behind. Stretch upward as you breathe in, and move forward as you find extra length with the out breath. Eventually your chest will touch your thighs and in that position the spine can go on lengthening with every exhalation.

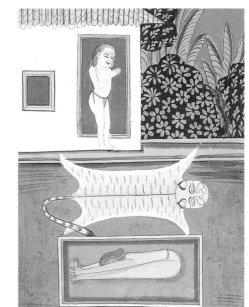

Practice makes perfect. The cliché applies as much today as it did to a seventeenth-century yoga practitioner.

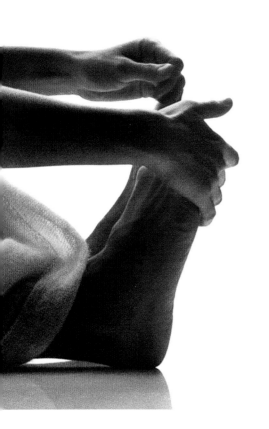

Day after day let the yogi practice harmony of soul: in a secret place, in deep solitude, master of his mind, hoping for nothing, desiring nothing.

BHAGAVAD GITA

PASCHIMOTTANASANA
Forward Bend

KURMASANA
Tortoise

The tortoise's apparent calm and quietness is felt in mind as well as body once you can envelop yourself in this asana with ease.

Kurmasana is dedicated to one of the ten incarnations of Vishnu, Maintainer of the Universe. Vishnu turned himself into a giant tortoise and dived to the bottom of the ocean to retrieve important treasures of the gods lost in a great flood. There are three stages to this asana. First the tortoise is out of its shell with its front legs stretched ahead of it. In the asana the legs extend forward over the arms. In the second stage, the palms turn up and the arms come around the sides of the body to stretch out behind. The last stage, Supta Kurmasana, is called sleeping tortoise because it resembles the tortoise when it has drawn its head and limbs into safety and quiet beneath its shell. And yes, once this asana has been mastered, it is a quiet resting pose which soothes the nerves and tones the spine and abdominal organs. It is one of the sacred asanas, the withdrawing of the head

and limbs symbolizing the withdrawal of the senses and emotions.

You start sitting with the legs wide, dropping the torso down between bent knees. Then you scoop the arms under the knees, opening your chest out toward the floor so that the arms can flatten out to the sides and the heels push along the floor in front of you until the legs are as straight as possible. In Supta Kurmasana, you rotate the arms and take them around the back of your body, aiming to clasp them across your back. Then you cross your ankles over your head, tucking the back of the neck into the little space under the crossed ankles. This is not an easy pose if the hamstrings, the lower back, or the hips are tight, but it is one that can respond fairly quickly to practice. The real tortoise has developed special muscles to help it breathe, as its shell prevents it from expanding its chest.

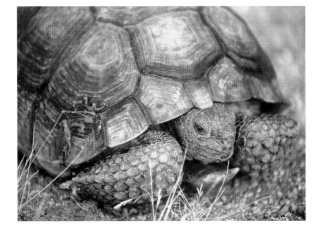

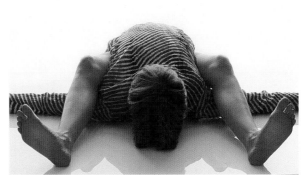

When in recollection he withdraws all his senses from
the attractions of the pleasures of sense,
even as a tortoise withdraws all his limbs,
then his is a serene wisdom.

BHAGAVAD GITA

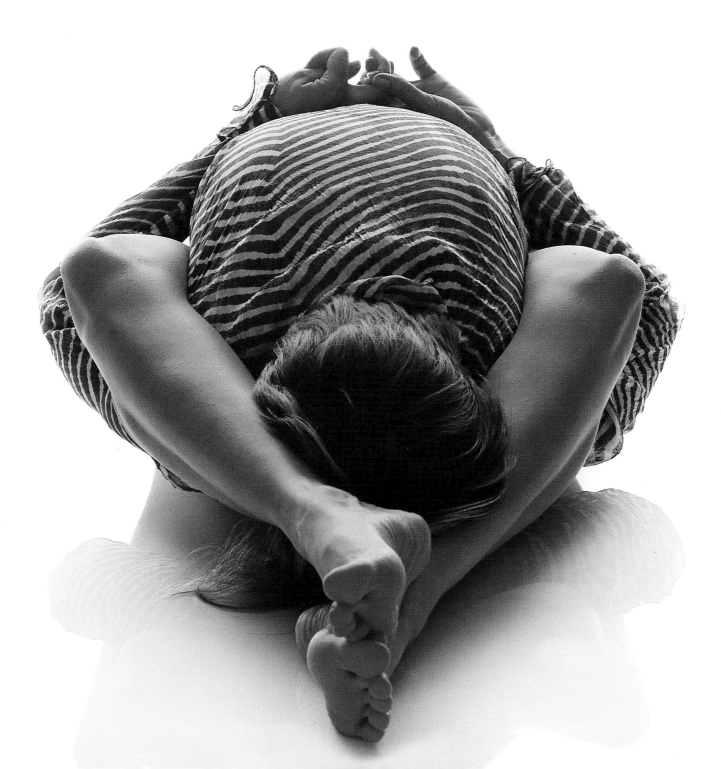

There is a Light that shines beyond all things on earth, beyond us all, beyond the heavens, beyond the very highest heavens. This is the Light that shines in our hearts.

CHANDOGYA UPANISHAD

Pindasana is a very gentle pose that many people use between more strenuous asanas in their yoga practice as a resting position. The figure of the Muslim lady praying in the privacy of her garden terrace in what we recognize as Child's pose is also an exquisite gesture of humility and reverence so universal that every culture may recognize and respond to it.

Pinda means embryo in Sanskrit. When someone curls up in the embryonic position we understand this as a desire for protection and safety. This gives the spirit of the position but doesn't explain why Pindasana is such a good pose to rest in. When we look at photographs of embryos in the early stages of development, we see that the spine is the first recognizable part of the fetus to develop, and it does so in this lengthened position, curled around the front of the body, protecting the vital organs as they develop. Many children and even adults continue to sleep in this position, as it is a wonderful way to stretch the back safely and comfortably. As there is little tradition in the West for sitting or kneeling on the floor after childhood, Pindasana can initially be difficult because of stiffness in the hips and knees. This problem does not present itself so much in the East where, even now, sitting on the floor, both kneeling and cross-legged, is part of the culture. For all Muslims, this prostration is one stage in a whole sequence of prostrations for the daily prayer. The Prophet Muhammad exhorted his followers to perform the prayer, with its sequences of standing, bowing, kneeling, and prostrating, not unlike yoga's Salute to the Sun sequence, five times every day. He, too, must have understood that for the mind and spirit to be truly healthy it had to inhabit a healthy body.

In Child's pose it is easy to follow the breath. Watch your back ribs expand as you inhale, and feel your neck and shoulders relax. With each exhalation your spine grows longer as gravity pulls the heavy hips down toward the floor and you begin to let go.

Left. This nineteenth-century painting from Lucknow shows a gentle-woman performing one pose in the sequence of prostrations that make up the Muslim prayer. A universal gesture of humility, it bears a striking resemblance to Child's pose, itself part of the prayer sequence in yoga called Salute to the Sun.

PINDASANA
Child's Pose

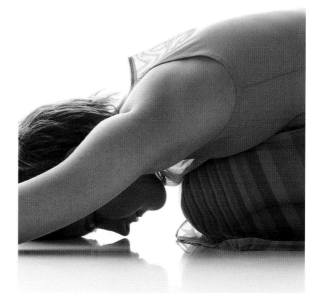

BADDHA KONASANA
Bound Angle or Cobbler's Pose

As with so much in yoga, the simplest things are the most difficult to master.

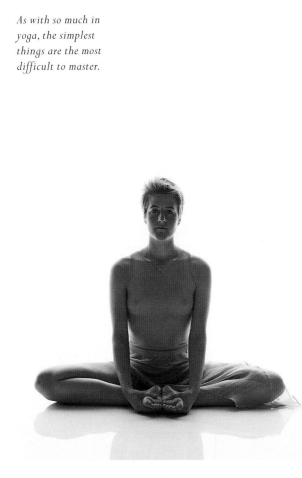

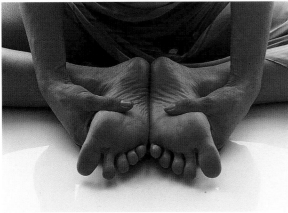

This is one of the most ancient asanas of all, shown in seals from the Indus Valley dated around 2000 B.C.E. In the West we often refer to it as Cobbler's pose, or Tailor's pose, since shoemakers, tailors, tent-makers, and other craftsmen can be seen sitting like this in markets all over the Orient as they sew away, day in and day out, in their workshops. In Sanskrit, *baddha* means caught or bound, and *kona* indicates an angle.

In Baddha Konasana the heels push together and the thighs turn out. The hips can then relax, letting the pelvis take its own weight to the ground. People with stiff hips find it difficult to do this without slouching the back, in which case it is best to work at this pose sitting with the back supported against a wall. Once you are comfortable in Baddha Konasana, open the feet like a book and turn the soles to face the ceiling, as if you wanted to read what was written on them.

Eventually, the base of the pose is so well rooted that the legs become light enough for the hands to lift the feet up off the floor, bringing them to touch the chest quite easily. To have flexibility in the feet is of paramount importance in yoga. If the feet are stiff and closed, the function of the knees, hips, and ultimately the lower spine will all be compromised. It is also impossible to find good roots in the standing poses without feet that are alive and supple.

Baddha Konasana stimulates the blood circulation in the whole of the pelvic region. It helps keep the kidneys, the prostate, and the urinary tract healthy. For this reason it is particularly recommended for those with urinary disorders and for pregnant women. It is also one of the poses to practice if Lotus is difficult, as it opens the hips and groins without hurting the knees.

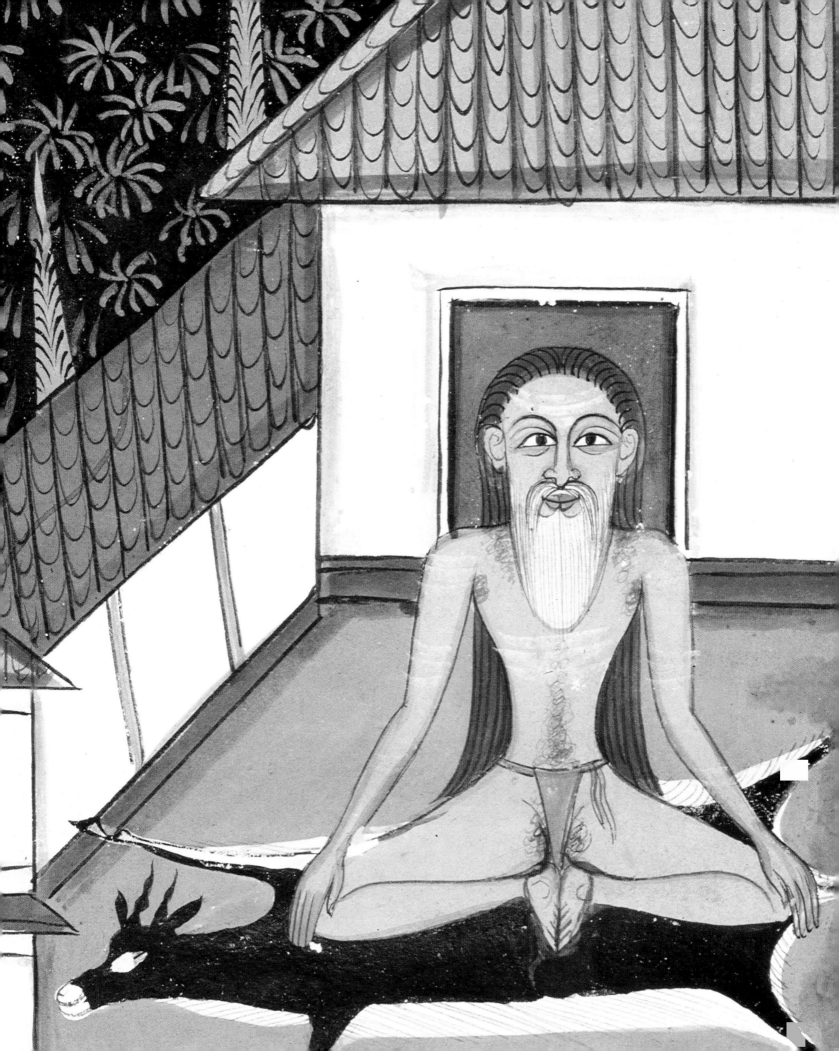

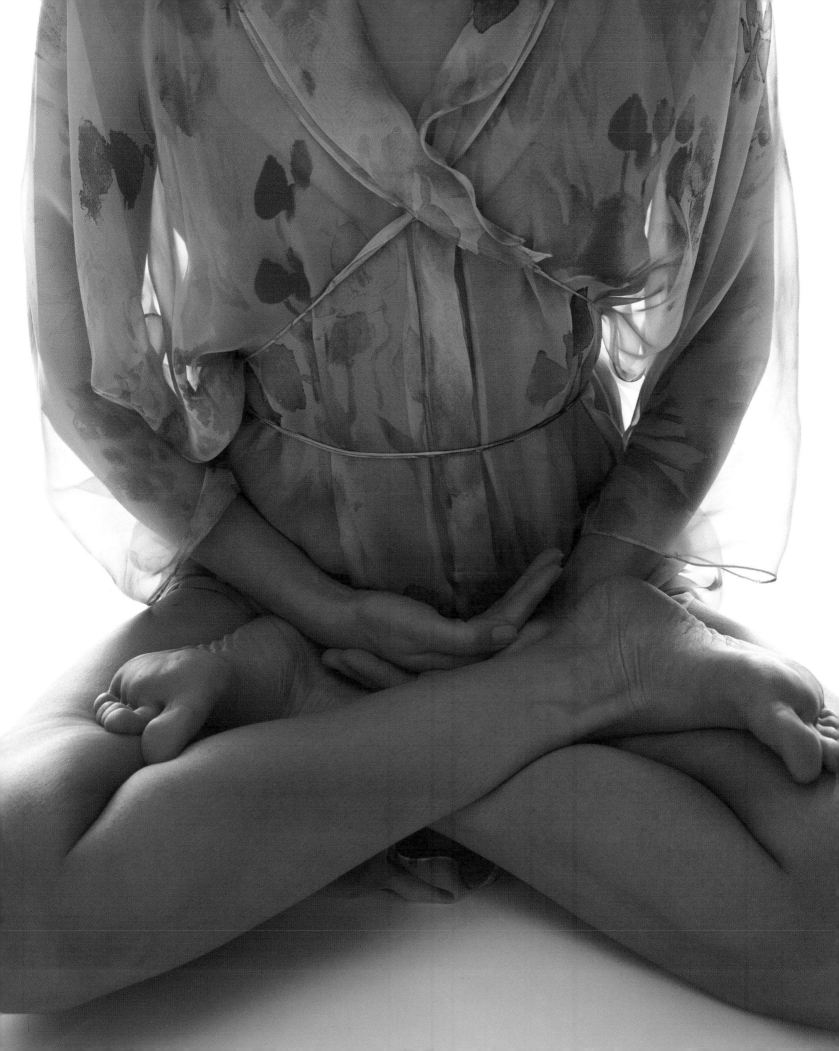

Lotus

Most of the innumerable pictures and sculptures of the Buddha and other sages meditating show them in this classic sitting pose. If you can do it, it is the best way to sit for meditation and pranayama, since the pose is so naturally rooted and stable that the spine has no choice but to lengthen upward away from this base.

The unfurling petals of the lotus flower have long symbolized the experience of deep meditation, in which the layers of consciousness peel open in the mind. This must explain why this pose, most conducive to meditation, is so-named. But we might imagine as we do Lotus that the body, too, is opening up like the lotus flower, from a strong, serene core.

According to the esoteric teachings of Hatha Yoga, the aim of all yoga practice is to awaken the divine cosmic energy, symbolized by the serpent, Kundalini, coiled dormant at the base of the spine, and to channel that energy up through the six chakras that lie along the *susumna nadi*, the central channel along the axis of the spine. When the awakened creative force reaches the seventh chakra at the crown of the head, it is said to bring about a transformation of consciousness. So intense is this spiritual experience that many gurus, sages, and psychoanalysts have warned of the dangers of attempting to awaken the kundalini. But one does not have to go to these extremes to enjoy the physical benefits of sitting in Lotus. A word of warning, however: If you have stiff hips, which many people in the West suffer from, you are most unlikely to be able to get into this position without damaging your knees. Never force your way into Padmasana. It takes some people years of working on the hips, knees, and ankles in other positions before their joints are flexible enough to do it in safety and comfort.

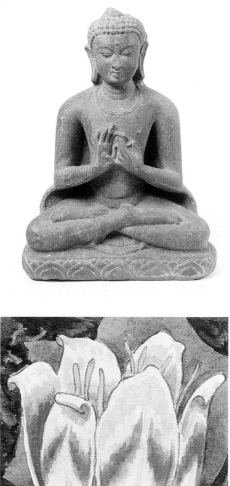

The true Lotus pose combines core strength with serenity. The latter doesn't come without the former.

PADMASANA
Lotus Twist

Once you can do Lotus, it has many variations to play around with. It can be done standing on your head, in Shoulderstand, bending forward, lying on your stomach or back, and lifted into an arm balance. It can also be the starting point for a simple twist that, because the hips are anchored down by the crossed legs, allows the spine to twist from a very firm base in a gentle and effective way. Someone who has been practicing this for a long time will have flexible feet, which, because they are no longer stiff in the pose, can be used as levers to keep the hips down and facilitate the movement.

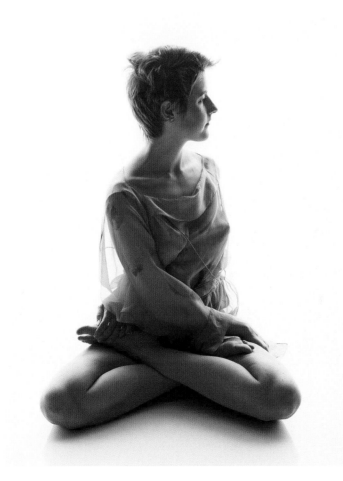

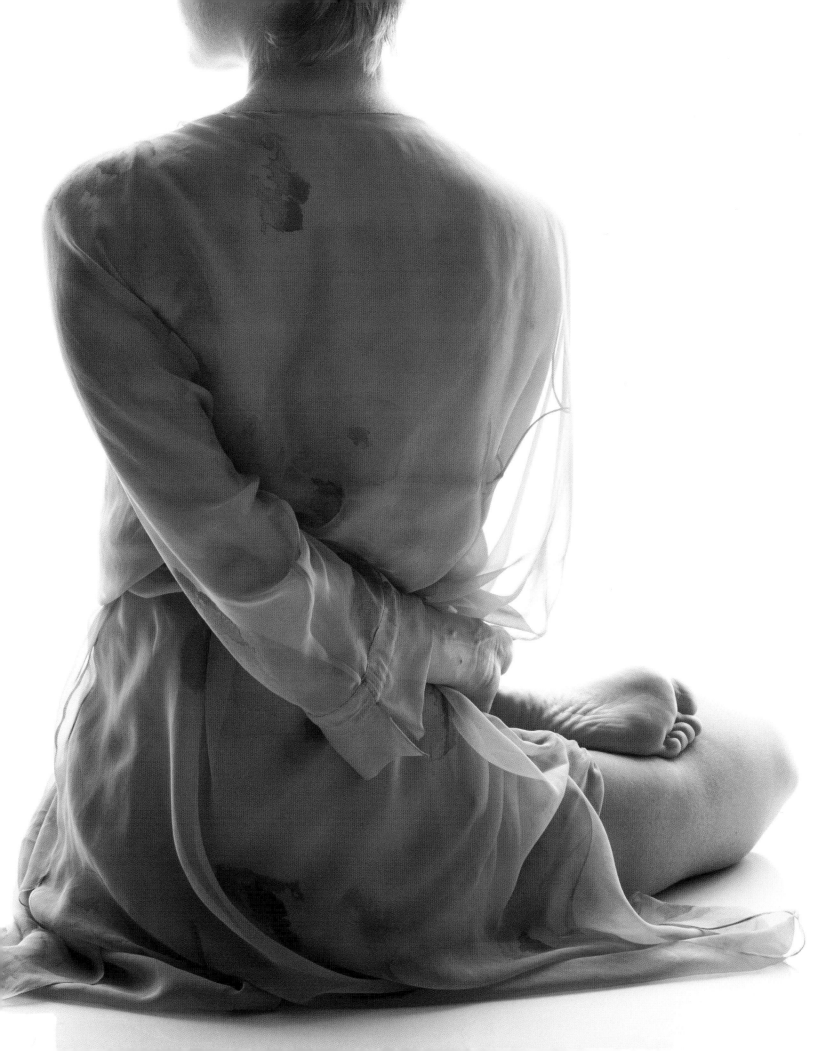

Surya Namaskar is the ancient ritual of saluting the sun. One of the best known yoga sequences, it combines the benefits of all the asanas, pranayama, and bandhas. There are many variations of Salute to the Sun, but basically it comprises twelve poses, one for each month of the year, which flow from one into another in a dance of breath and movement to honor the morning sun.

Starting in Tadasana, Mountain pose, with the palms together in Namaste, the gesture of greeting and respect, you breathe in and lift your arms above your head. Then, breathing out, you bow down into Standing Forward Bend, and inhale to take a leg back into Lunge. From Lunge, you hold your breath as you take the other leg behind you, and straighten both of them so that your body is suspended in Plank, with the trunk firm and the palms and toes touching the floor. Then you exhale and take the body down into Full Prostration. This is the midpoint of the sequence, and a gesture of total submission and humility, with feet, knees, chest, hands, and chin all in contact with the ground. With the end of that exhalation, you draw up into Cobra,

where you breathe in. On the next exhalation you move into Dog, then swing the leading leg forward again into Lunge with an inhalation. With the next out breath, bring the back leg forward as well, and open your knees so that you find yourself back in Standing Forward Bend. As you take your last breath in, your heels go down and you come back into Tadasana with your arms raised above your head, to draw a great circle that brings your hands back into Namaste. Now you are ready to start all over again, leading, of course, with the other leg. Only when you have done the whole sequence twice, leading with each leg, have you completed one cycle of Salute to the Sun. Traditionally this is done twelve times at dawn.

Some people consider Surya Namaskar the complete yoga practice. With its controlled breathing, backbends and forward bends, invigorating and calming poses, it is certainly a balanced cycle. This is the sequence to perfect if you want to give yourself a good aerobic workout, as long as you take care to keep in rhythm with your breath as you speed up.

SURYA NAMASKAR
Salute to the Sun

What soul was his, when from the naked top
Of some bold headland, he beheld the sun
Rise up, and bathe the world in light.
"THE EXCURSION." WILLIAM WORDSWORTH

SAVASANA

Corpse

Savasana should be done at the end of every
practice. It is not as easy as it looks to surrender
yourself utterly to the floor and lie relaxed but
alert to the quiet vibrations of your body.
It is amazing how often people find excuses for
not staying for this bit at the end of a class – falling
asleep is the other common way people avoid it.

The deep relaxation that comes after an
intelligent asana and pranayama practice is both
refreshing and invigorating; it also ensures that you
don't rush from the more active part of yoga asana
practice into the frenzy of everyday life, which
could turn your practice into nothing more than
just another form of exercise.

In some ways Savasana is a precursor to meditation,
as it requires you to renounce the fidgets and fusses
of the body and mind and give yourself up to your
breathing. As you lie flat on your back on the floor,
your whole body learns to relax, with the pull of
gravity taking you further into the ground. If your
mind wanders you can bring it back to focus on the
easy rhythm of the breath.

Lying upon one's back on the ground at full length like a corpse is called Savasana.
This removes the fatigue caused by the other asanas and induces calmness of mind.

HATHA YOGA PRADIPIKA

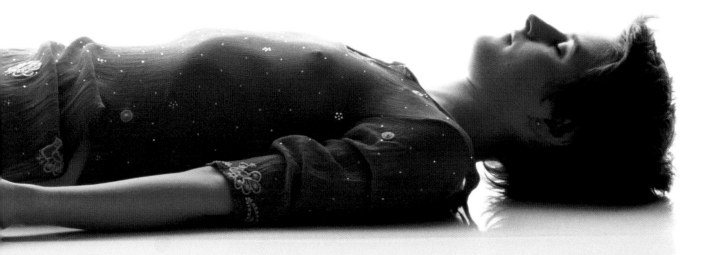

The breath is the intelligence of the body.

T.K.V. DESIKACHAR

PRANAYAMA IS THE CONTROL OF THE BREATH so that it may tune the body, calm the mind, and ultimately be used as a route to deeper levels of consciousness. *Prana* means many things in Sanskrit – it is not just the word for breath, but also life-force, cosmic energy, air, and strength, as if yoga does not distinguish between the breath of the individual and the pulsing energy of the cosmos. The English language, too, links the concept of the breath with the mystery of the human condition – the word "inspiration" is another word for inhalation.

Our breath is intimately linked with our state of mind. It gets shorter when we panic, higher up in the chest when we're stressed; it is fitful when we are anxious, becomes even and quiet if we are calm and serene, and appears almost to disappear altogether when we are concentrating hard. If fear can make us pant, it makes sense that we should be able to master a panic attack by consciously deepening and quieting our breathing. Patanjali said that the practice of pranayama developed the powers of concentration and clarity of thought. Others have interpreted this on a deeper level. In *Yoga, Immortality and Freedom*, Mircea Eliade points out how such control of the breath could give one an opportunity to experience "in perfect lucidity, certain states of consciousness that are inaccessible in a waking condition… By reaching the rhythm of sleep through the practice of pranayama, the yogin, without renouncing his lucidity, penetrates the states of consciousness that accompany sleep."

PRANAYAMA

Coming at the same subject from a slightly different angle, Andrew Weil, in his bestselling *Spontaneous Healing*, says, "if breath is the movement of spirit in the body, then working with breath is a form of spiritual practice. It is also one that impacts health and healing because how we breathe both reflects and influences the state of the nervous system."

But if pranayama is a route to spiritual or mystical experience, it is also, and perhaps more important for most of us, the key to putting our feet firmly on the ground and finding a secure base from which to walk confidently through life. Our first breath is drawn at the very moment when our body feels the pull of gravity for the first time. From that instant, our breath is forever bound up with our sense of our physical self, and our feeling of security. "Breathing is the key to grounding," says Mary Stewart. "Every exhalation brings you down to quiet and rootedness. Breathing practice should be simple, still, and quiet. It's about reality, not dreams. It is not about a mystic experience. It shows you how to be in the moment."

The life of the yogi is traditionally measured not by the number of years he lives, but in the number of his breaths. In simple terms then, by controlling the rhythms of the breath and learning to extend them, one may grasp the secret of longevity. Indeed, many of the best known gurus of the modern age have been extremely long-lived; Krishnamacharya, one of the fathers of modern yoga, lived for 101 years and was teaching six weeks before his death in 1989, and Vanda Scaravelli was ninety-three when she died in the first year of this millennium.

The mind may also be calmed by expulsion and retention of the breath.

PATANJALI

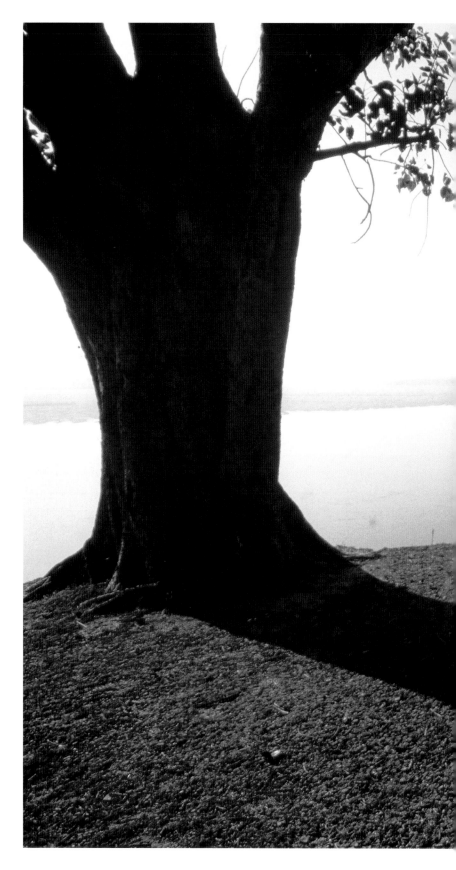

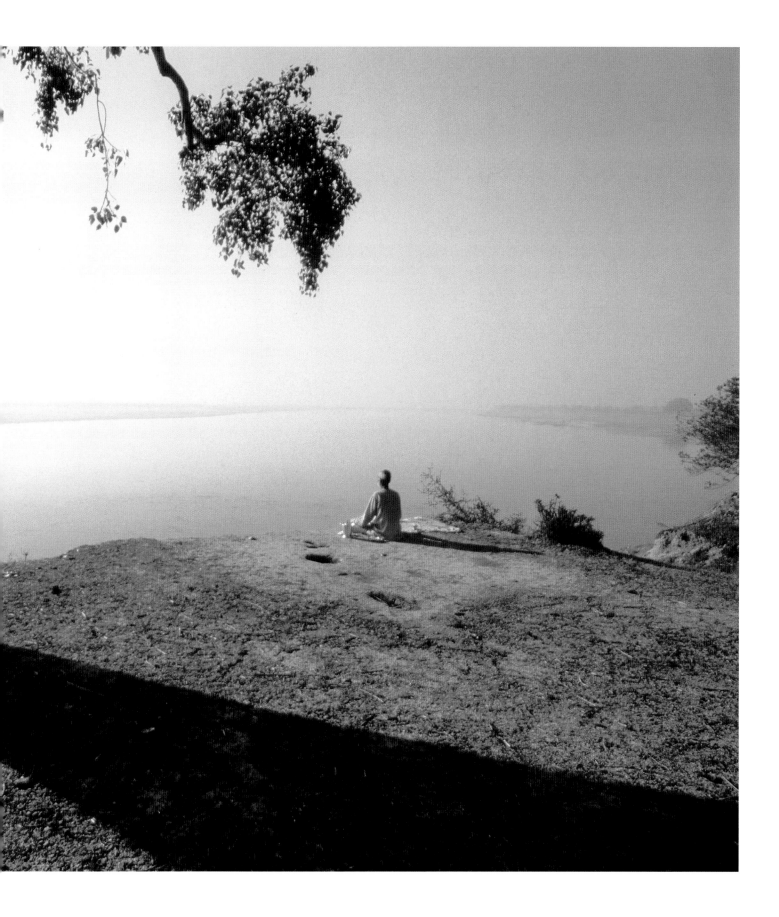

KRIYAS, BANDHAS, & MUDRAS ~

The *Hatha Yoga Pradipika* identifies six cleansing processes, or kriyas, as well as bandhas and mudras, all of which aim at detoxifying and strengthening the body in preparation for pranayama practice.

KRIYAS ~ Kriyas are cleansing rituals. They were originally devised to cure sickness. Although not widely practiced in the West – and most should not be attempted without medical supervision – simple instructions, like those for clearing the nasal cavities with a steam inhalation containing a few drops of eucalyptus oil and ghee, are a safe, useful, and universal remedy for sinusitis, colds, coughs, and bronchitis. Anyone who has covered their head with a towel over a steaming bowl of Friar's balsam or essential oils will know this to be a simple but effective therapy. More complicated kriyas, none of which should be undertaken without the supervision of an experienced teacher, include: Dhauti – swallowing a sterilized muslin cloth and then regurgitating it to cleanse the stomach; Nauli – a rhythmical contraction of the abdominal rectal muscles that stimulates peristalsis; Trakata – cleansing the eyes by focusing on a selected object and gazing at it without blinking until the eyes tire or water; Neti – two ways of cleansing the nostrils, one with lukewarm salt water, and the other by inserting a long thread into one nostril, training it down the back of the throat and pulling it out through the mouth; Vasti – washing out the intestines by drawing water up through the rectum; Kapalabhati – a breathing technique for clearing stale air out of the lungs.

BANDHAS ~ The bandhas are muscular locks that occur naturally in the body when one has learned asanas with proper control of the breath. They protect the body from the increased pressures in the abdominal and thoracic cavities caused by pranayama, and help to redirect the flow of prana, or vital energy, that has arisen in the body from pranayama. It can be helpful to know how they work, but they must never be forced.

Jalandhara Bandha ~ This is a chin lock where the neck elongates and the chin fixes neatly into the notch between the neckbones. It is developed particularly through the practice of Shoulderstand. It regulates the flow of blood to the heart and to the brain, and it massages the thyroid and parathyroid glands.

Uddiyana Bandha ~ Most people have seen photographs of this dramatic pulling in of the abdomen, in which the internal organs are pushed back toward the spine and up toward the diaphragm. Contemporary pictures of the pop star Sting doing this pose with accompanying text about his ability to have sex for five hours are very misleading. Uddiyana actually happens quite naturally when one breathes deeply in a position that allows the spine to lengthen. It is particularly evident in Headstand, in which gravity draws the internal organs higher up anyway. This bandha tones and massages all of the internal organs, and is very good for the heart. According to the *Hatha Yoga Pradipika*, it makes the "great bird of prana" fly up the main channel of nervous energy situated inside the spinal column, and is so rejuvenating that, as Iyengar claims, "he who practices it as taught by his guru or master becomes young again," confirmation that the correct practice of yoga can lead to a youthful appearance and the prospect of longevity.

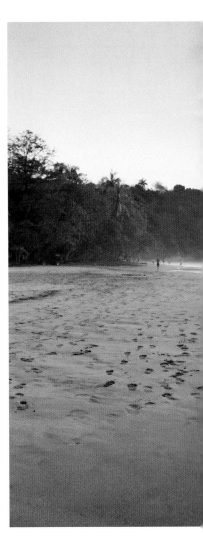

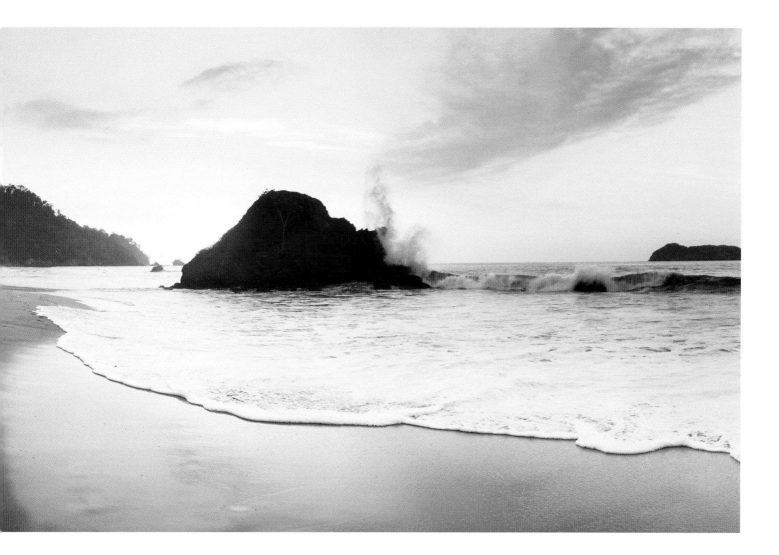

The inexorable ebb and flow of the tide is like the natural rhythm of the breath.

Mula Bandha ~ *Mula* means root, origin, or foundation. The Mula Bandha is the pelvic-floor exercise every woman is instructed in before and after the birth of a child to strengthen muscles stretched by birth. These muscles form a sort of hammock beneath the trunk, supporting the internal organs and linking the pubis with the sitting bones with the sacrum and coccyx. The whole region between the anus and the scrotum or vagina and pelvic floor is lifted up as the lower abdomen draws in toward the back of the waist on the exhalation.

MUDRAS ~ In Sanskrit, *mudra* means gesture. In the practice of yoga, mudras help

the action of the bandhas. They complete circuits of energy by bringing attention to a certain point in or on the body. The quiet placing of the palms of the hands on the back in Shoulderstand is an example of a mudra, and as with all mudras, it should be a profoundly calming and centering gesture. Two other mudras most commonly identified are Jnana Mudra, which is joining tips of the index fingers and thumbs, leaving the other three fingers open – traditionally used in meditation as it symbolizes the union of the individual soul with the Infinite; and Kechari Mudra, which involves curling the tongue back so that its underside touches the roof of the mouth.

THE ART OF BREATHING ~

What distinguishes ordinary shallow breathing from deep abdominal breathing is the role played by the diaphragm, the body's largest and perhaps most underrated muscle. As you inhale, the diaphragm contracts, reducing the pressure in the thorax as it flattens down and drawing air into the lungs. As you breathe out, the diaphragm relaxes and moves back up into its domed position in the chest, reducing the available space in the thorax and expelling the air from the lungs. Many adults are shallow chest-breathers rather than the deep abdominal-breathers we were designed to be. When the diaphragm is properly engaged in breathing, it acts like a pump stimulating the whole abdominal and portal circulation.

There are three functions of breathing that we learn in pranayama: inhalation, *puraka*; exhalation, *rechaka*; and retention, *kumbhaka*. Inhalation enlarges the chest cavity and fills the lungs with fresh air, supplying the body with oxygen and stimulating the whole system. Holding the breath increases the carbon-dioxide level in the blood, raises the internal temperature, and plays an important role in increasing the absorption of oxygen. During exhalation the diaphragm returns to its relaxed, domed position, and as it does the stale air from the lungs, full of toxins and impurities, is pushed out.

You can help to engage your diaphragm by drawing in your stomach muscles as you breathe out. Then you will find a moment at the end of each exhalation, as the diaphragm reaches its point of relaxation, when the spine lengthens naturally. But you have to be quiet and attentive to observe it. And when you find it, enjoy it. Don't rush to snatch at the inhalation. Wait for it to come in of its own accord and at its own speed, filling your lungs and widening the back of your body. It can be helpful to think of calm waves lapping onto a shore while you breathe. On the exhalation, visualize the pull of the tide drawing the water back out. Then the waves pour back across the sands as you breathe in, inevitable and inexorable. Even the noise that calm waves make as they ebb and flow across sand or shingle are not unlike the sounds of quiet, deep breathing.

For the diaphragm and other respiratory muscles to be able to function freely, one must be sitting correctly. The spine and its muscles must balance themselves with the movement of the diaphragm, so that the lower vertebrae draw downward with the exhalation, allowing for a release in the spine. The pelvis must not be tilted either back or forward, allowing the spine to hold itself effortlessly, each of its four curves balanced easily with the other three, and the head carried weightlessly at its point at the top, with the shoulders relaxed and the chin tucked in.

The Lotus pose is the classic position for sitting to breathe or meditate, precisely because it takes one naturally into this balanced position. But the sculptures of the Buddha sitting in Lotus make it look deceptively easy, which, of course, it isn't. Many people work at Padmasana for years before they can sit in it comfortably for any length of time. Alternative positions then are Vajrasana, Baddha Konasana, or even sitting in an upright chair, with both feet firmly on the ground. Whichever way you sit, the same rules apply. When you inhale, the shoulders have a tendency to rise up, so be careful to keep them soft, and use the exhalation to let them drop again, and feel soft and long in the back of the neck.

Breathing is so bound up with the essence of how we are that it is not something we can change either by force of will or with any speed. The harder you try in pranayama, the more elusive the breath will become. In the end, we all learn that we can only change the breath by giving it attention, by watching it.

SOME PRANAYAMA EXERCISES ~

"As lions and tigers are tamed very slowly and cautiously so should prana be brought under control very slowly in gradation measured according to one's capacity and physical limitations. Otherwise it may kill the practitioner." This rather dire warning from the *HathaYoga Pradipika* addresses an important point. Pranayama is a powerful tool and should not be taken lightly. There is nothing wrong with teaching yourself the principles of simple deep breathing from a book, but all of the other pranayama exercises should be learned from a qualified teacher.

Ujayii ~ Simple Deep Breathing ~ This is the simplest of the pranayama exercises, and one that it is safe to teach yourself. Done either lying on your back with your knees bent, or sitting, Ujayii is a slow rhythmical inhalation and exhalation without effort. Breathe out, draw your belly in, and watch the spine lengthening and the hips and shoulders releasing as you relax at the end of the exhalation. Do not take the breath in, but wait to receive it in its own time. Slowly and surely, with each cycle of the breath, the body will adjust itself as the spine moves and finds its own equilibrium with the breath. In this way, Ujayii teaches the perfect sitting position. If it helps to make the length of the breathing regular, count smoothly and evenly as you breathe, and over time it will get deeper and slower. Don't expect the same from your breathing every day, though. Your breath is the first function of the body to be affected by how you are feeling.

Kapalabhati ~ Cleansing Breath ~
One of the kriyas, Kapalabhati is a method for clearing the sinuses. It cleans the respiratory tract and nasal passages and helps to eliminate gases from the stomach and intestines. It also revitalizes the mind and improves concentration. A Kapalabhati breath is a sharp contraction of the abdominal muscles, forcing stale air out through the nostrils, followed by the immediate relaxation of the abdominal muscles, drawing fresh air in. It is a powerful method of breathing which should not be done for too long. If you feel remotely high after practicing it, you will have been hyperventilating. It should not be practiced by people with eye or ear complaints, by those with high or low blood pressure, or by pregnant women.

Kumbaka ~ Restraining the Breath ~
To put the body into a position that any normal person would find impossible and then hold it – in other words to perform an asana – has been described as the first indication of yoga's aim to transcend the human condition. When the same analysis is applied to pranayama practice, Kumbaka, the retention of the breath, is the ultimate, for it amounts, in Mircea Eliade's words, to "the 'refusal' to breathe like the majority of mankind." In Kumbaka we do not, of course, stop breathing altogether, but we hold the breath for a measured length of time, in a strict ratio with the length of the inhalation and the exhalation.

Bramari ~ Exhaling with a Vibration ~
Bramari, also known as the humming or buzzing breath (the sound that is made on the exhalation is like the buzzing of a bee), is one of the few pranayama exercises that is safe to practice alone. As you breathe out, you make a buzzing noise with the vibration of the lips. As you get quieter and the buzzing becomes more internalized, you can feel the vibration deep in your breastbone, and then traveling through the body down the spine. It is a calming exercise, and it can be helpful for people beginning to learn pranayama, as the sound distracts one from too many imperatives about how one should and should not be breathing.

And when the body is in silent steadiness, breathe rhythmically through the nostrils with a peaceful ebbing and flowing of breath. The chariot of the mind is drawn by wild horses, and those wild horses have to be tamed.

SVETASVATARA UPANISHAD

MEDITATION is a poor translation for what the Chinese call "sitting still doing nothing" (*ching-jing-wu-wei*). Taoists and Buddhists believe that every human is born with a precious pearl of original spirit deep inside the core of his or her being. This precious pearl is a mirror that reflects the entire universe. In India there is Samadhi meditation, "stilling the mind," which is common to Hinduism, Buddhism, and Jainism. It is considered an essential part of spiritual practice because it provides the possibility to channel all one's mental energy and direct the mind in a single, pointed way.

Every culture has its answer to meditation; to just sit and "be" is a human need that we ignore at our peril. Contemporary Western life appears to be unconducive to this urge; our over-developed analytical approach to reality and experience makes it difficult for many of us to get a grip on the concept of meditation, let alone practice it. Nevertheless, there is a strong tradition of mysticism and the contemplative life in Western Christianity, and today more and more people in the Western world are taking up regular meditation, as they find that their achievement-orientated, materially focused lifestyles have not brought contentment. It is this letting be, allowing our thoughts and anxieties to quiet, that we want desperately to learn.

If you practice yoga asanas and pranayama, sooner or later the attentiveness and quietness it brings lead inevitably to the deeper concentration of meditation. Of Patanjali's eight "limbs" of yoga, the last three concern meditation; they are known as the "inner path," distinguishing them from the first five, which include, of course, asanas and pranayama. These last three are *dharana*, concentration; *dhyana*, meditation; and *samadhi*, illumination.

DHARANA ~ The first of the three stages of the inner path is learning to sit and focus the attention on the moment. This is difficult. When we first sit to meditate, even to find a minute or two of quiet without the usual mental chatter appears to be impossible. Obsessively, the mind seems to return to the problems of the day, fantasies about the future, memories or regrets about the past. And we are so caught up in these things, and so used to it, that we can sit, outwardly quiet, for a full five minutes before even realizing that we've been racing all over the place in our mind. Just sitting in silence can be immensely hard, lonely, and even threatening for some people.

In dharana, we make use of tools the mind can hold onto in order to learn the profound concentration required for meditation. These tools include mantras, yantras, and the simple process of following one's breathing. Some teachers recommend specific times of day for practicing meditation, but the biggest battle is to find the discipline to set aside a regular time every day, whatever time of day that might be. Begin slowly, giving five minutes, twice a day, to sitting and breathing. With commitment, this will grow organically into longer and longer periods until you may arrive at a place where you can sit in meditation for half an hour or longer without any awareness of the passing of time. The secret of meditation is to commit your time to daily practice. You cannot learn meditation by reading a book about how it will change your life.

Mantras ~ In his book *The Heart of Creation*, the Benedictine monk John Main says, "In meditation, by learning to say your mantra, you learn to trust, you learn to be. Indeed, the joy of meditation is that it is a celebration of being, a celebration of sheer joy in receiving your life as gift, and doing what Blake called 'kissing the joy as it flies.' Prayer is not possessing, not controlling, but

sheer celebration of being. We come to this celebration because the meditation leads us to centeredness, to the still point. In each person there is a still point that is me but is not exclusively me. What you will learn from your own experience in meditation is that there is only one center, which is the center in all centers. This is the understanding we come to in meditation, again out of our own experience, of the profound unity of being, the unity that is in us and the unity in which we have our being."

Traditionally a disciple is given his or her mantra by a teacher. It is a private and sacred communication between the two, chosen to reinforce the chain from teacher to disciple down the generations. The disciple is supposed to take this mantra for life and repeat it endlessly. A mantra is repeated from the beginning to the end of the period of meditation, first so that the mind has something to come back to when it starts wandering, and then, once that has been mastered, so that the vibrations of the word become rooted in the unconscious. The mantra is repeated in rhythm with your breathing and also, supposedly, with the beating of your heart. T.K.V. Desikachar explains in his book *The Heart of Yoga*: "You must understand the word mantra correctly. It is not a Hindu symbol but rather something much more universal: It is something that can bring a person's mind to a higher plane. Sound has a lot of power; the voice has a tremendous influence. Just think about how an orator can capture an audience just by the way he speaks. In our Indian tradition we have made use of these qualities of sound. In India we use mantras because, by virtue of their religious tradition, they mean something to many people. But I would never use a mantra indiscriminately. We can always work within an individual's tradition. What is universally true is that sounds can have a powerful influence on us."

I shut my eyes in order to see.
PAUL GAUGUIN

Right. So complete is the expression of peace on the face of this sixth-century marble buddha from the northern Qi dynasty of China, that as we contemplate it we, too, are drawn closer to the realm of meditation. Did the sculptor intend to make of his work of art a tool for meditation, like a mandala or yantra?

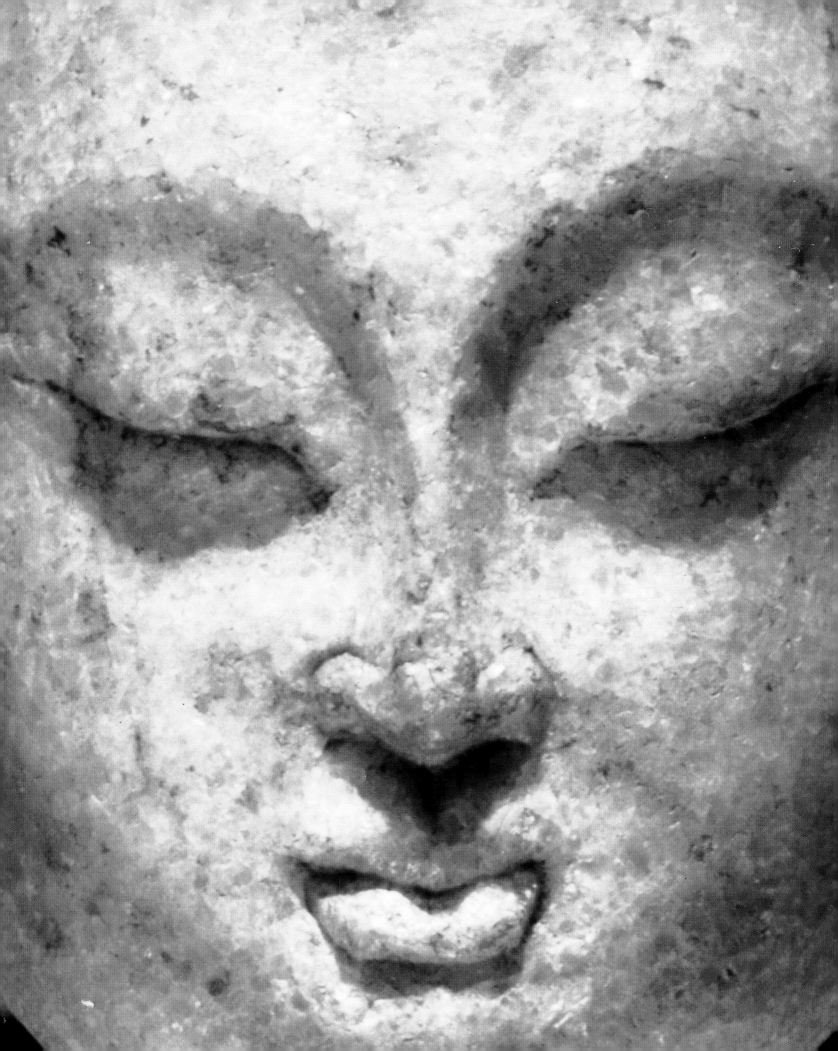

Most rituals designed to alter our state of consciousness make use of some sort of sound, whether chanting or drumming. Indeed, the Jesus prayer is one practiced in the Orthodox Church in a way not dissimilar to a mantra.

Of all the mantras, AUM, or OM, represents everything for the Hindu: It is the sound of creation, the beginning and end of everything, and the most ancient word known for God. Throughout the history of mankind, it has been God's name that is called upon in times of crisis and inspiration. Take this line from The Book of Proverbs: "The name of the Lord is a strong tower: The righteous runneth into it and is safe." The *Mandukya Upanishad* says, "AUM stands for the supreme Reality. It is a symbol for what was, what is, and what shall be. AUM represents also what lies beyond past, present, and future."

Yantras ~ The yantra is a sort of visual mantra, intricate but hypnotic, that can be looked at and internalized for meditation. A yantra, known in the Tibetan-Buddhist tradition as a mandala, represents in either geometric or figurative forms the different layers of consciousness and the principle of creation, much as AUM does in sound terms. Indeed, the written symbol of AUM is also used as a yantra, the three shapes symbolizing the creation, maintenance, and destruction of the universe. Jung recognized the mandala as one of the archetypal symbols, representing the human striving for wholeness. This fits in with Fosco Maraini's description of the mandala: "A mandala is essentially an ideal construction; it can be traced in the sand, created by means of colored powders or flowers on a plain surface, painted as a mural, or even created three-dimensionally in sculptures or buildings (pagodas/temples). Certain towns have been planned on the basis of a mandala – Beijing and Kyoto for instance."

Again we can find parallels in other traditions. Take, for example, the use the Orthodox Church makes of icons.

DHYANA ~ Having mastered the concentration of the mind, one reaches a point of unwavering stillness, where the mind cannot be distracted. This is dhyana, meditation.

SAMADHI ~ Samadhi is the goal of the yogi's quest. At the peak of meditation, the practitioner passes into the state of samadhi or transcendence, beyond consciousness into bliss. In this state the yogi is totally aware and alert but at the same time not part of this world. This state could be translated as ecstasy, but that would be dangerous. The tools of meditation are powerful, and, used with the wrong intentions, can be destructive – think of the chanting of the mob and the evil it can engender, and know how controlled breathing patterns can upset the delicate internal balance of the body. If you approach meditation looking for weird experiences, or with ambition for power, you are more likely to find your way to psychosis than to a place of clarity and equilibrium.

Right. This mandala is also a diagram that represents the universe and its orbits.

The peace of God which passeth all understanding.
PHILIPPIANS

Yoga is the control of the thought waves of the mind.
PATANJALI

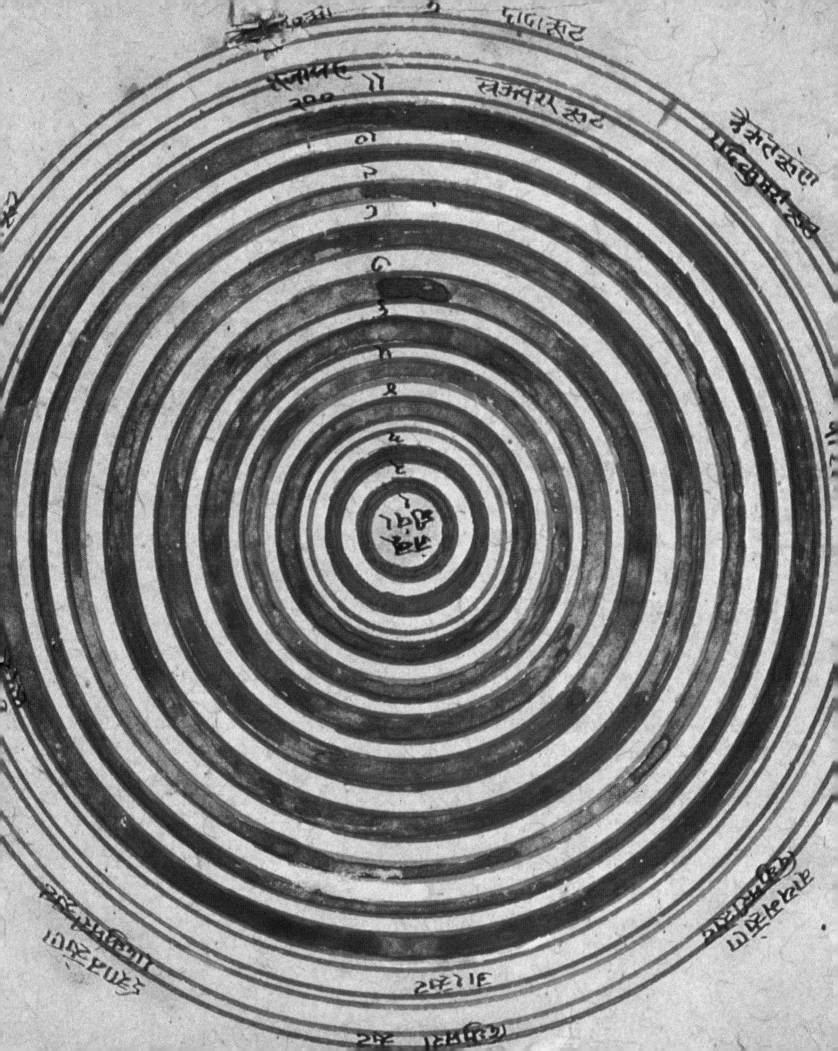

BACK TO THE ROOTS OF YOGA

If I were asked under what sky the human mind has most deeply pondered over the greatest problem of life, and has found solutions to some of them which well deserve the attention even of those who have studied Plato and Kant — I should point to India. And if I were to ask myself from what literature we who have been nurtured almost exclusively on the thoughts of Greeks and Romans and of one Semitic race, the Jewish, may draw the corrective which is most wanted in order to make our inner life more perfect, more comprehensive, more universal, in fact more truly a human life, again, I should point to India.

MAX MÜLLER

FEW COUNTRIES CAN MATCH the scale and diversity of India and no other country has its religions so intertwined with every aspect of life. India is a vast subcontinent of contrasts, at once crowded and remote, luxurious and squalid, with flat plains and majestic mountains, palm-fringed beaches and holy rivers. It is a noisy, eccentric, colorful, mystical land full of temples, sacred sites, ritual, haunting music, heroes and demons, ascetics and seekers. It is the birthplace of two of the world's greatest religions, Hinduism and Buddhism, and one of its quietest, Jainism. More than seven hundred million people in India practice Hinduism, but India is also still home to millions of Muslims, to a large community of Christians, and to one of the few remaining communities of Parsis, who practice Zoroastrianism, as well as to the comparatively recent religious tradition of Sikhism.

In Indian mythology, the Himalayas have always been the abode of the gods, and here, perhaps more than anywhere, in the shadow of these mountains that lie between India and Tibet, the complexity and diversity of India's religious culture persists like nowhere else. Among remote mountain ranges, fertile valleys, and jungles is the Kathmandu valley – the playground of the gods. This is just one of the places that Hindus and Buddhists alike have christened *pithasthan*, the "power places." These are places where geomantic significance combines with myth, legend, and superstition to create focal points of powerful magnetic energy, never more tangible than on ritual festive days where temples pulsate with chanting, dancing, and the wilder ceremonies that still involve sacrificial offerings.

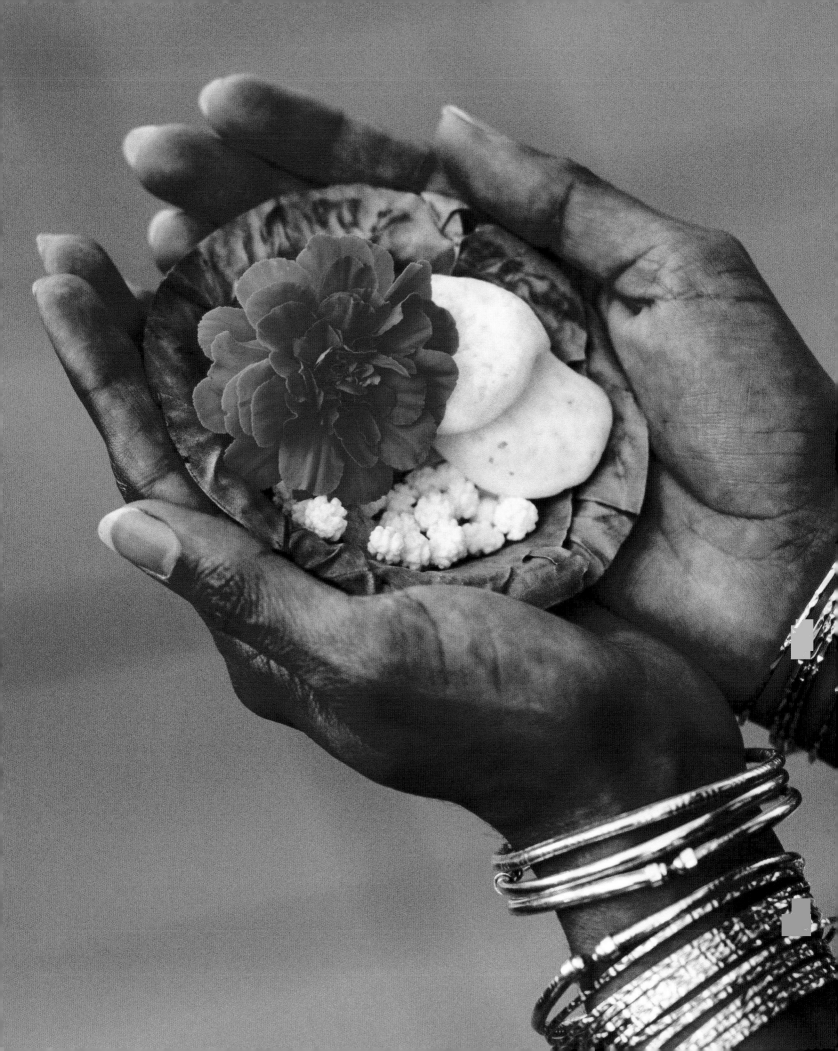

In these areas unhewn rocks and boulders suggest the shapes of familiar deities; the elephant-headed Ganesh, or Shiva's lingam. And these become places of pilgrimage and worship. Temples, pagodas, monuments, and shrines mark residences of the gods between the peaks of the snow-covered mountains. Thousands of devout pilgrims from Buddhist and Hindu traditions alike have always traveled to these special places for spiritual renewal and realization.

Hinduism is a complex and contradictory religion, with its multiple gods and many forms of worship that vary greatly from region to region. But essentially all Hindus believe in *Brahman*, the One. Everything that exists emanates from Brahman and will ultimately return to it. The multitude of gods and goddesses (some estimate numbers of deities in the millions) are all manifestations of the phenomenon of Brahman. Hindus commonly believe in an earthly cycle of rebirths; you are born again and again in a condition dependent on the karma you acquired in previous lives. Living a *dharmic* life – dharma signifying appropriate behavior – will enhance your chances of being born again into a higher caste and a better life. Bad behavior might result in rebirth in animal form, but it is only as a human that you have the opportunity to gain enough self-knowledge to escape the cycle of reincarnation and obtain *moksha*, or liberation. A fundamentalist would say moksha is not an option for Hindu women. They can hope only to be born the next time round as a man. The hardline also states that to be a Hindu you must be born in India of Hindu parents, there is no other way. The way to self-knowledge was written down in sacred texts including the *Bhagavad Gita*, which is still required reading for most Indian school children. The emphasis is on the study and practice of yoga, meditation, and devotion.

For four thousand years India has withstood invasion, famine, persecution, and political upheaval. Modern India is still a country of infinite variety as modern technology and change are incorporated into the fabric of society, and yet the age-old truths, the holistic point of view, and the essence of Indian philosophy is as present as ever, to the endless and increasing fascination of the Western world.

The philosophy of India is extremely complex and has been studied and analyzed in depth and with great difficulty, since there is no certainty as to the names of those to whom many writings are attributed, nor any exactness regarding the dates of composition. Even the task of translating Sanskrit and Pali concepts into intelligible Western language is something that arouses controversy among scholars, not least because there are six basic systems of Hinduism – and innumerable subsystems – four chief schools of Buddhism, two schools of Jainism, and so on, all using some of the same language in different contexts. The task of unraveling all this is way beyond the scope of this chapter, which aims only to place yoga in its historical and conceptual context.

Indian philosophy concentrates largely on man's spiritual destiny, which is why it is so bound up with Indian religion, often blurring the boundaries between the religions, particularly between Hinduism and Buddhism. In thousands of years of Indian scriptures passed down over the centuries there are many references to yoga as a path toward the Truth. The development of Indian belief systems may be roughly and approximately divided into four major periods of development: the Vedic Period, *c.* 2500–600 B.C.E.; the Epic Period, *c.* 600 B.C.E.–C.E. 200; the Sutra Period late B.C.E. and early C.E.; and the Scholastic Period, which some say continues to this day.

It is not enough to know the truth; the truth must be lived.
The goal of the Indian is not to know the ultimate truth
but to realize it, to become one with it.

SARVEPALLI RADHAKRISHNAN

Right. Often in India the sheer vastness of a crowd can remind one of the awesome history of this continent's innumerable gods, rituals, and faiths. Here, hundreds of thousands of Hindus converge in Kerala for the annual festival of Trichur Pooram.

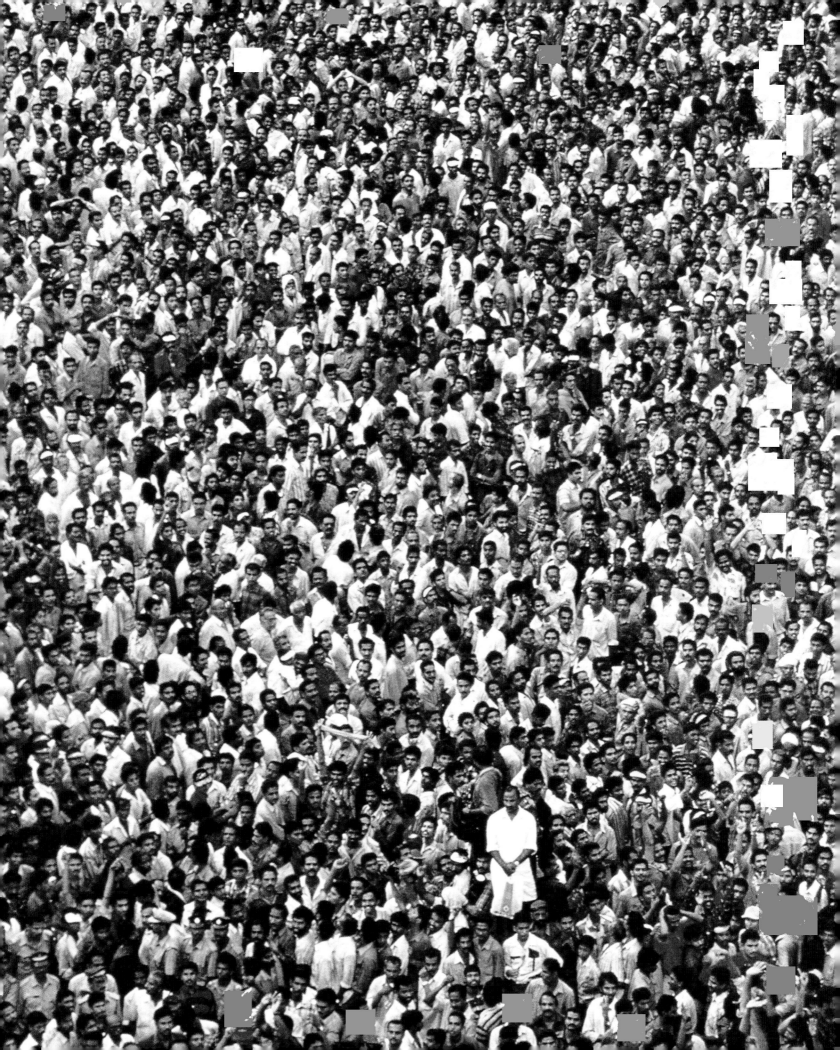

The most beautiful and most profound emotion we can experience is the sensation of the mystical. It is the sower of all true science.

ALBERT EINSTEIN

THE VEDIC PERIOD, which dates back to at least 2500 B.C.E., is the era when Aryan (from a Sanskrit word meaning noble) tribes came down from Afghanistan and Central Asia to India and began to filter into northwest India and make it their new homeland. Eventually these tribes controlled the whole of northern India as far as the Vindhya Hills, and many of the original inhabitants of these lands were pushed south. The invaders brought with them their gods of fire and battle, Agni and Indra respectively, as well as their meat-eating tradition. It was during this time that the Hindu scriptures, the Vedas, were composed and the caste system became formalized, distinguishing the Aryans from the indigenous Indians whose lands they had conquered.

The word *veda* means wisdom, and the four hymns known as the *Rg Veda*, *Yajur Veda*, *Atharva Veda*, and the *Sama Veda* are important because they constitute the beginning of Indian philosophy as we know it. The Vedas were composed long before writing was introduced into India. The poems and songs reflect the different religious and philosophical ideas current during that age. Each of the Vedas contains four sections, including hymns and prayers and discussions of the significance of sacrificial rites. Here man is looking at the world in awe and wonder. He feels the life he lives, and prays for victory while he venerates nature's living powers; the sun, the moon, and the elements of earth, water, fire, and air. The early hymns muse on the creation of the world, representing the older philosophies that were bound up with gods and goddesses such as Aditi, who signified the boundlessness of the universe and infinity, and later, Varuna, who represented cosmic order.

THE FIRST SONGS: THE VEDAS

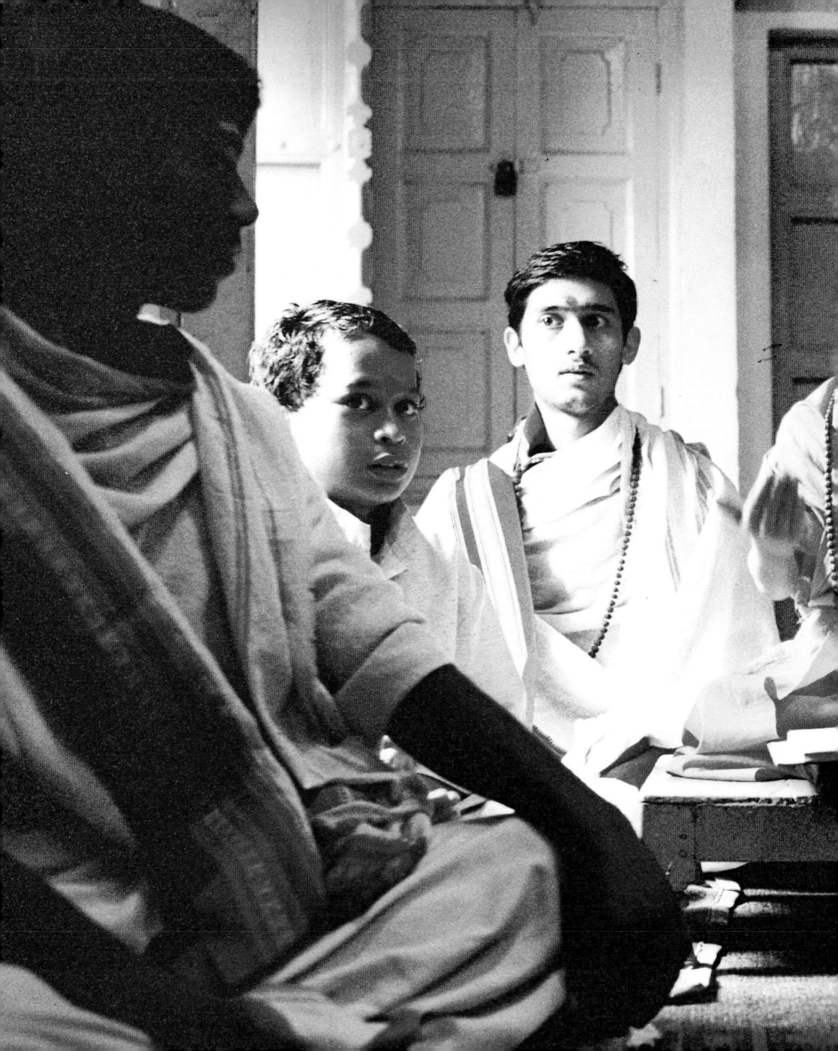

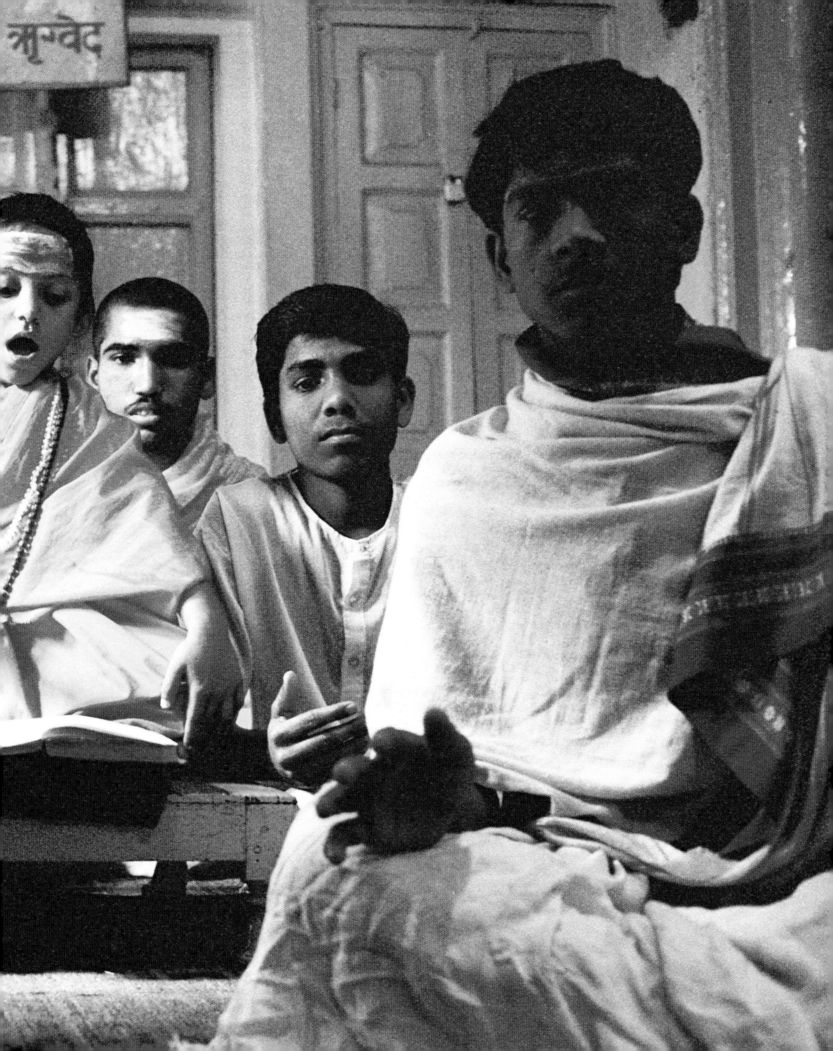

The whole universe is ever in this power. He is pure consciousness, the creator of time; all-powerful, all knowing. It is under his rule that the work of creation revolves in its evolution, and we have earth, and water, and ether, and fire, and air.

SVETASVATARA UPANISHAD

Many other deities were named after natural phenomena – Indra and Agni as already mentioned, and other examples, such as Surya, the Sun god, and Prthivi, god of earth. Here was the first inkling of God as the creator of nature, and of nature as God itself. The *Atharva Veda*, with its spells and sacrifices, is said to contain the beginnings of Indian medical science, but it is the *Rg Veda*, which comprises more than a thousand hymns, that is considered the most important of the four. This is because it represents the earliest evidence of an evolution in religious consciousness. It is the work of priests in awe of the immensity and mystery of the universe – by contrast with the later crystallization of thought set down in the Upanishads, which were the work of philosophers.

It is thought that a long period of time elapsed between the compilation of the many hymns of the *Rg Veda*. The later ones signify a development of thought from polytheism to monotheism. Gradually it seemed to make more sense that there should be one God rather than many, but even this single great Being was questioned in the writings: "One and another shall say, There is no Indra. Who hath beheld him? Whom then shall we honour?" Still later Vedic philosophers were not entirely satisfied with the idea of one God and went on searching for what they considered the absolute truth. Finally the doctrine of the impersonal, unknowable One, Brahman – the source of the universe, and *Atman* – the soul, or the Self, overtook previous thinking and this, as well as the concept of birth and rebirth in successive lives after death, became the theme of the latest writings of the Vedic period, the Upanishads.

If the Vedas preceded the Upanishads, they also set the tone for them. The word Upanishad is derived from *upa*, meaning near; *ni*, down; and *shad*, to sit, evoking the way in which students would gather around the teacher to learn his words of wisdom by heart. In the Upanishads, hymns to the gods and goddesses are replaced by a search for the truth of the creation of all things: "For fear of whom fire burns, for fear of whom the sun shines, for fear of whom the winds, clouds, and death perform their offices?" asks the *Tattrirya Upanishad*.

The Upanishads' rather more sophisticated themes reflect on the mystery of death and emphasize the oneness of the universe. They explore the seminal idea that Truth is within us: *Tat tvam asi*, "That Thou art," a thesis pounced on by the Theosophists. They lay emphasis on right action and wisdom and condemn the lazy and narrow-minded path as the route to dissatisfaction — there is an almost practical aspect to them, in some ways heralding the tone of the *Bhagavad Gita*. They speak of the importance of an inward journey of self-realization. The means of achieving the ultimate reality and immortality are only to be found through discipline and perseverance and an inward journey. Here the word yoga is mentioned as the way forward: "When the five senses and the mind are still, and reason itself rests in silence, then begins the Path supreme. This calm steadiness of the senses is called Yoga," *Katha Upanishad*.

The *Mandukya Upanishad* explores the famous theory of the four states of consciousness — waking, dreaming, sleeping, and a deep-sleep state of all-knowing, higher consciousness — all of which is familiar ground to those studying Transcendental Meditation today. It is this discourse which explains the power and mystic symbolism of AUM, Hinduism's most venerated sign: "AUM, this syllable is the whole world. The past, the present, the future — everything is just the word AUM."

The names of the sages who wrote the Upanishads are not known. Eleven of the songs were later interpreted by the sage Shankara, an original thinker whose writings form the basis of Vedantic teachings. The dates of the Upanishads are difficult to determine, but they are thought to have been composed around the eighth and seventh centuries B.C.E. They form the basis of ideas later developed into the six orthodox systems of Hinduism — one of which was yoga — and of non-Brahmanic religious systems like Jainism and Buddhism that were to emerge after the Epic period.

Should you really open your eyes and see, you would behold your image in all images. And should you open your ears and listen, you would hear your one voice in all voices.

SAND AND FOAM, KHALIL GIBRAN

When all desires are in peace and the mind, withdrawing within gathers the multitudinous straying senses into the harmony of recollection. Then, with reason armed with resolution, let the seeker quietly lead the mind into the Spirit, and let all his thoughts be silence.

BHAGAVAD GITA

THE EPIC PERIOD, starting roughly in 600 B.C.E. and going on until about 200 C.E., gets its name from the two great epic writings of the period. They are the *Mahabharata*, of which the *Bhagavad Gita* is one book, and the *Ramayana*. These two tales are a fascinating potpourri of history, mythology, politics, philosophy, and theology, and they demonstrate a popularization of the way that philosophy and religious doctrine had begun to be represented and assimilated. Inevitably, there are many variations of both stories, as part of their appeal was in the way that they could be adapted in the telling, to make them up-to-date and relevant to the audience for whom they were being performed. The *Mahabharata* is a very political work, and thought to have been a manifesto of sorts for the ruling and warrior classes, since it focuses on the exploits of their favorite deity, Krishna, who embodied power and was able to legitimize right action. Certainly on the face of it, the conversation between Arjuna and Krishna in the *Bhagavad Gita* appears to condone, even encourage, political war. The *Mahabharata* is also thought to be the world's longest literary work, eight times longer than the Greek epics the *Iliad* and the *Odyssey* put together.

The ancient art of storytelling has to a large extent been replaced today by film and television, and Peter Brook's adaptation of the *Mahabharata* into a film, famous as much for its epic length as anything else, is an elegant symbol of this. Nevertheless, the drama and compelling power of the stories themselves are not lost on most Indians, who are still brought up on the *Bhagavad Gita*, and eighty million of whom tuned in to the *Mahabharata* when it was serialized by Indian State television in the 1980s.

*Krishna talking to
Arjuna in a scene from
India's great poem, the*
Bhagavad Gita.

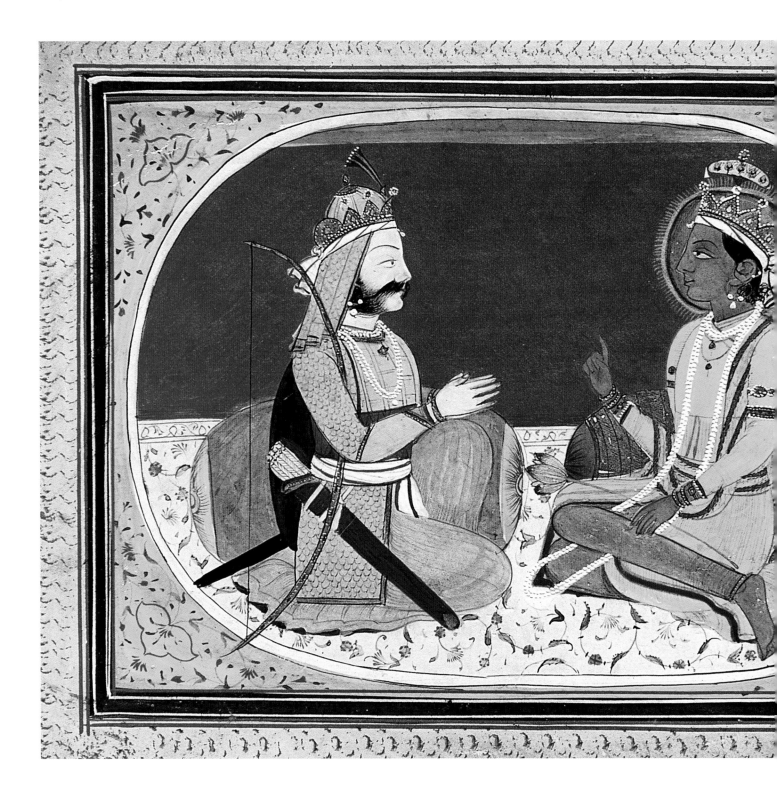

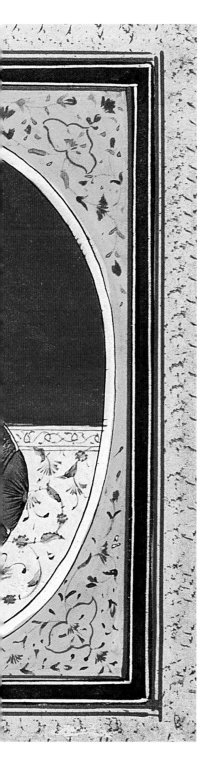

Whoever knows himself knows God.

THE PROPHET MUHAMMAD

The *Mahabharata* tells the story of a battle between rival kings, and while it symbolizes the struggle between the forces of good and evil, there is much evidence to suggest that it is based on historical fact. Nevertheless, Sanskrit literature never strove for historical accuracy, substituting for it romance, idealism, and practical wisdom, as well as spiritual knowledge. The epics provided a context in which ideas could be represented by characters, making the spiritual messages within them more easily understood and remembered.

It comprises eighteen books and one hundred thousand couplets. The *Bhagavad Gita*, often called the fifth Veda, is just one of these books. Its name translates as "song of god," and it is one of the most important and authoritative scriptures of yogic philosophy, as well as having had a great influence on the development of Indian thought and life. Unlike the great war that is the subject matter of the rest of the epic, the *Bhagavad Gita* is a conversation between Krishna, an incarnation of Brahman, appearing in human form to Arjuna, his son and pupil, and Arjuna. In the Upanishads, Krishna and Arjuna are represented by the more abstract notions of Brahman as Absolute Reality and Arjuna as the inner truth of Atman, the soul or the Self.

Famous warriors are assembled on either side of a battlefield when Arjuna, the greatest archer in the world, suddenly wakes up to the fact that he is pitted against teachers, friends, and relatives, many of whom he is likely to kill. He becomes fearful and anxious and, threatening to pull out at the last minute, asks Krishna, his teacher, to explain how the evil consequences of war can be justified: "Shall I kill my own masters who, though greedy of my kingdom are yet my sacred teachers?" Krishna's answer to this is summed up in these lines: "When a man sees that the God in himself is the same God in all that is, he hurts not himself by hurting others: then he goes to the highest Path."

"In the *Bhagavad Gita*," argues Juan Mascaro, the Cambridge academic who famously took twenty years to translate it, "Arjuna becomes the soul of man and Krishna the charioteer of the soul who shows him how right effort leads to Nirvana." This is a battle for the kingdom of heaven, which is also the kingdom of the soul.

During the eighteen chapters that make up this spiritual discourse, Krishna leads Arjuna through his doubts, one after the other; his fears of mortality, decisions on what action he should take, the importance of having a pure heart in the approach to all things, and the explanation of yoga. Three key themes reoccur again and again, namely *jnana*, meaning the light of knowledge; *bhakti*, meaning love or devotion without desire; and *karma*, which refers to life and right action. These have come to represent three of the four paths of yoga, the observation of each and all of which lead to yoga. The fourth path, *raja*, is the most elusive to definition. It is mentioned in the *Bhagavad Gita*, but it is not as pivotal to the narrative as the other three, and it only becomes significant to the development of yogic philosophy with the advent of Patanjali.

Another important theme in the *Bhagavad Gita* is that of contemplation, which distinguishes it from the Vedas and Upanishads, in which emphasis is placed on the significance of external ritual. By the time of the epic period, it is the inner spiritual life that is held up as the conduit to joy. Nevertheless, the *Bhagavad Gita* is far more of a practical guide as to how to lead life than any writing that went before it. Again and again we are told that through self-control and harmony, selfless work, and devotion we will find God or bliss or happiness or immortality or contentment: "A harmony in eating and resting, in sleeping and keeping awake: a perfection in whatever one does. This is the yoga that gives peace from all pain." The spirit of this message is a far cry from some yogis' interpretation of self-control, which leads them to eccentric and exhibitionist practices like hanging themselves out of trees from meat-hooks, lying on beds of nails, and holding their arms up in the air for years on end. The ultimate and enduring message of the *Bhagavad Gita* is one of hope.

For all its greatness, the *Bhagavad Gita* is just one, albeit superlative, example, of a wealth of philosophical material – and there were almost certainly more that didn't survive to the modern era – that was composed around this time. It was from these spiritual and philosophical visions, all developing side by side over centuries, that the five schools of orthodox Hinduism and the other, nonorthodox systems, namely Buddhism and Jainism, came to be formulated.

Spiritual poetry is common to many cultures. There is the Chinese Tao, the wisdom of Confucius, there is the sublime poetry of the Qur'an, the Psalms, and the Sikh writings, Buddhist incantations, and Shinto poetry. All of these

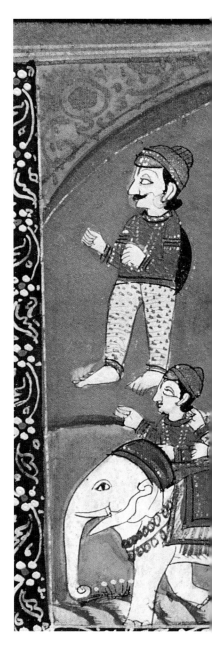

"Whenever his faltering mind unsteadily wanders, he should restrain it and bring it under self-control." The words of Krishna in the Bhagavad Gita *came to L. N. Agarwal's mind. But they were followed immediately by Arjuna's more human cry: "Krishna, the mind is faltering, violent, strong and stubborn; I find it as difficult to hold as the wind."*

A SUITABLE BOY, VIKRAM SETH

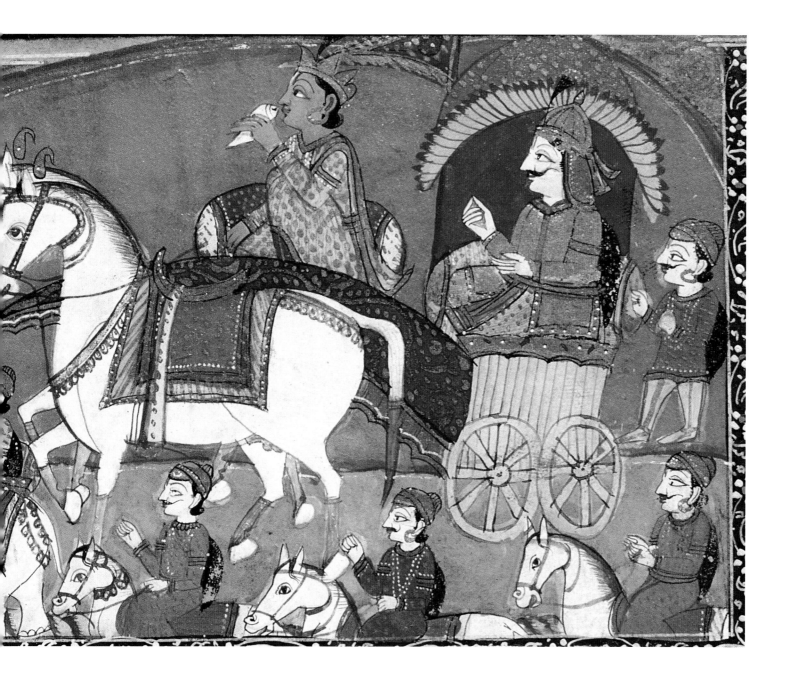

*Indian miniaturists
depict the symbolism
at the heart of the*
Bhagavad Gita, *where
Arjuna represents the
soul and Krishna is
depicted as his
charioteer, leading him
in way of right action.*

extol the glory of God, the beauty of the cosmos, and the value of unconditional love. The *Bhagavad Gita* and its story line are very much on a par with Christian and Buddhist thinking and seem extraordinarily modern. For this reason it has become a sort of Bible for many Indians, Buddhists and more recently Westerners, and is often quoted in modern literature today.

The *Ramayana* was composed in the early centuries C.E., and is believed to be largely the work of the poet Valmiki. It, too, is a long and winding story, with many variations, the bare bones of which are as follows. The childless king of Ayodhya calls on the gods to provide him with a son, and his wife gives birth to a boy, Rama, who is in fact an incarnation of the god Vishnu. The adult Rama wins the hand of the beautiful princess Sita in a competition and is chosen by his father to inherit his kingdom. But Rama's stepmother is not happy with this idea, wanting the kingdom for her son. She engineers that Rama, Sita, and Rama's full brother be sent into exile to live by their wits in the forest. This is when the many-headed demon king Ravana tries to seduce Sita, who refuses him. In a rage, he captures the princess and takes her off to his palace on the island of Lanka off the southern tip of India. Rama, assisted by an army of monkeys led by the monkey god Hanuman, eventually finds where Sita is held captive, and after a great battle in which his brother is mortally wounded, only to be saved by Hanuman, Ravana is overthrown and Sita rescued. In a dramatic and unexpected climax, Ravana recognises Rama as Vishnu and declares his wish to be killed by him, that he may become one with his god. Rama refuses to kill Ravana, and the former demon becomes Rama's devoted servant. They all return to Ayodhya where Rama puts poor Sita through a series of dreadful trials to prove that she was never unfaithful to him during her captivity. Eventually Rama is crowned king.

If the *Bhagavad Gita* is about the conflict between god and the soul, the *Ramayana* deals with the conflict of the Aryans with the natives of India, the land they have plundered and conquered, and the battle to integrate new cultures with indigenous ones.

Right. An illustration of the moment in the other great Hindu epic, the Ramayana, *when the monkey god Hanuman is caught on enemy territory by Ravana, the many-headed demon king.*

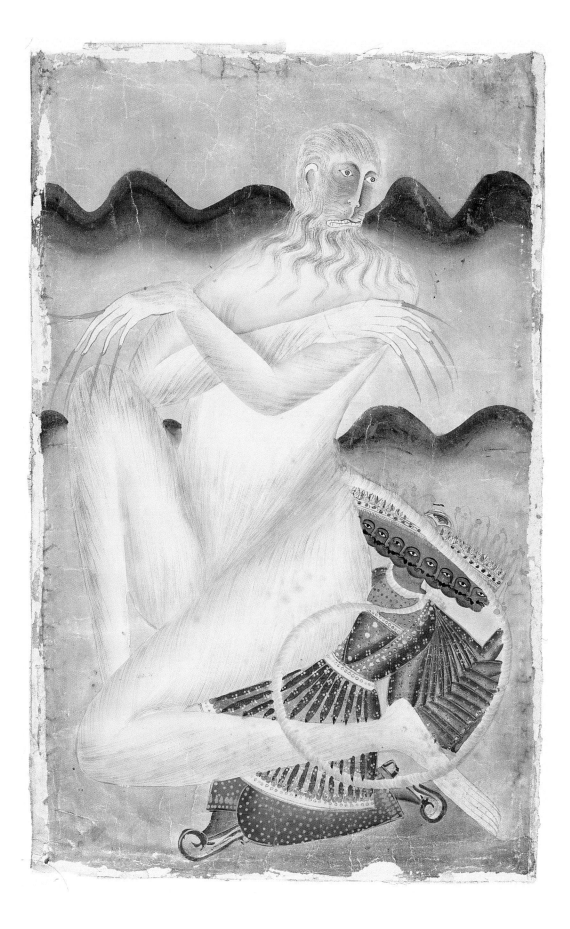

This sacred knowledge is not attained by reasoning, but it can be given by a true Teacher.

KATHA UPANISHAD

THIS PERIOD OF INDIAN HISTORY helps to define the extraordinary time of spiritual awakening just before and after the beginning of the Christian era, when Hinduism found its feet, and the unorthodox faiths came to be. Criticism and analysis began to take the place of poetry and religion, and philosophical and religious thought became split into six complementary systems of orthodox Hinduism. After the dramatic vision of the *Bhagavad Gita* and the polytheistic worship of the Vedas, this can be seen as a time where logic was used to set down current thinking on the nature of the origins of the universe and faith. The six systems of orthodox Hinduism, known as the Darsanas, were Nyaya, Vaisesika, Samkhya, Yoga, Purva Mimamsa, and Vedanta. All six systems were working on the same basis, attempting to explain the world and how to live properly within it, but they came at it from different angles. Meanwhile, the nonorthodox systems of Buddhism and Jainism were also taking hold.

THE FIRST INSTRUCTIONS: THE SUTRAS

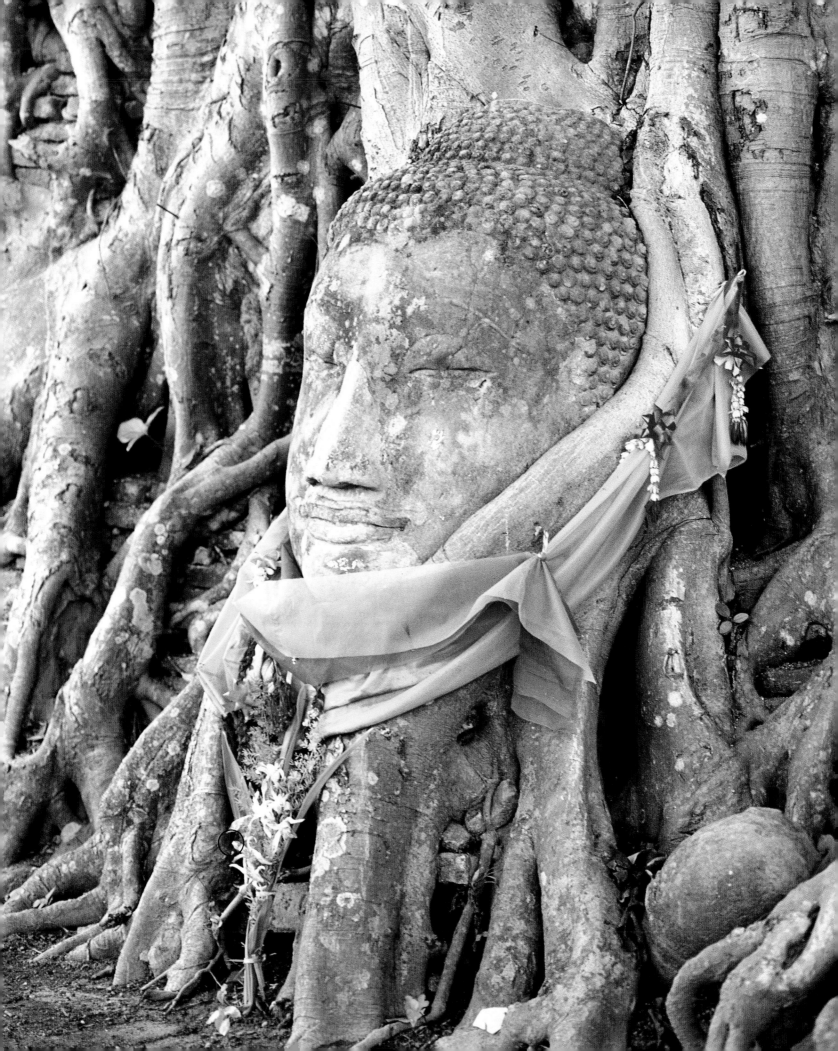

BUDDHISM AND JAINISM ~ The Buddha (which literally means awakened one) was born Siddhartha Gautama, the son of a king from the borders of Nepal and India. Renouncing his birthright of wealth and status at the age of twenty-nine, he became a wandering saddhu in search of enlightenment and finally achieved nirvana – the state of full awareness – at the age of thirty-five, at Bodhgaya. The Buddha's vision which, incidentally, renounced the caste system, was taken up in India for a thousand years and developed separately from the orthodox systems of Hindu thought and practice. Eventually Buddhism virtually died out in India while spreading to Tibet, Sri Lanka, Thailand, Korea, Indonesia, and China.

The Buddhist doctrine demands an eightfold path of morality, as does Patanjali's yoga system. The Buddhist goal was nirvana or the elimination of ignorance and selfishness. Right from the start the Buddha was something of a revolutionary and aimed at replacing the contemporary form of worship based on Vedic tradition, which was cosmos-orientated, with a practical quest for individual liberation. Living in the here and now was the crux of his teaching, and his rules for spiritual practice can be considered as the first known integral yoga system. To prepare the individual for transcendence, there are stages of behavior, of selfless service, unselfish thinking, and deep meditation in which the personality of the individual is left behind. A combination of right understanding, right thinking, right speech, right acting, right livelihood, right effort, right mindfulness, and right concentration leads to true knowledge and enlightenment.

Jainism did not accept the authority of the Vedas. The Jains believe that only by achieving complete purity of the soul can one attain liberation. Only by following the austerities of fasting, meditation, and living in solitude can one shed all karma. Fundamental to right conduct is *ahimsa*, nonviolence, and the Jain community was the first to make it a rule of life. Strict Jains maintain a bare minimum of possessions, which include a broom with which they famously sweep the path in front of them as they walk, to avoid stepping on any living thing, and a piece of cloth to tie over their mouths so that they cannot accidentally inhale even the smallest insect.

There are still some three million Jains in India, practicing their five virtues, of which nonviolence is the foremost and the others are truth-speaking, not stealing, chastity, and nonattachment to worldly things. These plus the three requisites for salvation – right faith, right knowledge, and right conduct (the five virtues) – are the Jain commandments.

Left. Nature and Nirvana. A head of the Buddha propped at the foot of a tree is entwined by the tree's roots. This embrace and the inevitable growth of the tree is leading them both upward toward the light.

THE YOGA SUTRAS OF PATANJALI ~ Yoga is one of the six systems of orthodox Hinduism and was set down as a Darsana by the sage Patanjali in his famous Yoga Sutras. These date from between 200 B.C.E. and 200 C.E. and form the basis of classical and Hatha Yoga. Nevertheless, looking at yoga today in its many incarnations, it is helpful to realize that some branches of yoga being taught are working from one or other of the six systems of orthodox Hinduism. For instance, the Siddha Yoga meditation teachings are based more on the beliefs of the Vedanta system than on the yoga. All six systems were laid out in the form of sutras, and many of them cover subjects taken up and discussed by the others. Yoga differs from some of the others in that it is not metaphysical. Patanjali's sutras were not theories up for discussion – they contain the essence of what was already an established discipline of ethical behavior, patterns already known through people's familiarity with the Upanishads and the *Bhagavad Gita*.

Sutra literature was written in the form of aphorisms: profound concepts encapsulated in concise sentences that may be accurately remembered and reproduced by learned and religious people. Their pithiness makes the sutras inevitably open to interpretation, which explains why the Sutra period was followed by a long period of commentary and analysis, known as the Scholar period. Indeed, the sutras are so concisely and densely expressed that it can be difficult to grasp the full sweep of their meaning without such commentary. They also represent the crystallization of the observations and gestations of many generations of thinkers, which is why it can be difficult to pin down their exact formulation. On top of this, there are cross references between the six Darsanas that were growing up side by side. The acceptance of the Vedas as the source for all six systems throws up several consistent themes.

EXPLORING A BELIEF SYSTEM ~ A thousand or so years before Patanjali's Yoga Sutras, the later Vedic poets had written about "the One," giving credit to some dynamic force or some form of consciousness that sparked off the creation of the world: "The sages' ray extended light across the darkness: But was the One above or was it under? Creative force was there, and fertile power: Below was energy, above was impulse. Who knows for certain? Who shall here declare it? Whence was it born, and whence came this creation?" (from the Creation Hymn of the *Rg Veda*).

In most mystical traditions, the "One" or "Cosmic Whole" is accepted as the first step in the creation of humanity. And whether the One is an outer force or an inner light, and whichever religious technique of prayer or contemplation is thought to be necessary to realize or make sense of the concept, it appears in Judaism, Christianity, and Islam as the one God, in Far Eastern religions as the Tao, and in the Indian tradition, represented here as the yogic vision, as Brahman.

Right. The sacred thread that the Brahmin wears across his torso distinguishes him from all other castes in orthodox Hinduism.

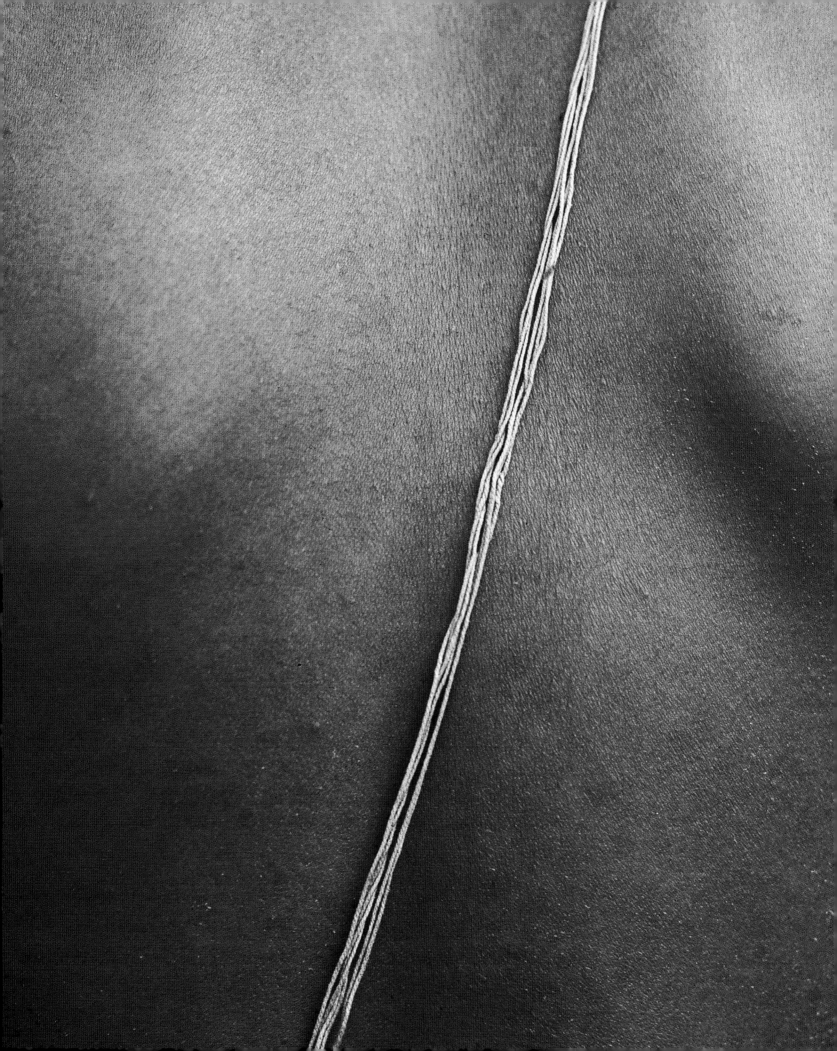

In the Samkhya Darsana, which is notable for its theory of evolution, all experience is based on the evolution of nature, or the matter from which the cosmos is made, known as *prakrti*, into pure consciousness, or spirit, known as *purusha*. In this model, purusha acts like a spectator or even catalyst to the force of prakrti, which is the protagonist of the action. In other words, evolution can only take place in the presence of consciousness. The yoga system accepts this theory of evolution but it brings God, or Brahman, into the equation, not as a creator but as a supreme being and the embodiment of all that is wise and good. By the time Patanjali came to chart the developments of these theories, the enquiry of the Vedas and the Samkhya theory of evolution had already been rejected by the Buddhists who maintained that the world was a continuous process brought about by mental will power with no beginning and no end. But in the yoga system, devotion to God is the route to perfection through the control of both the physical and psychic elements of human nature; as long as you are part of this world, you are always striving to integrate the two.

The concept of purusha is sometimes easier to grasp if it is interpreted as spirit and prakrti as matter. Indian imagery often represents purusha as the male principle – with the lingam, and prakrti as the female – the yoni. The aim of yoga is to create a union between these two, spirit and matter, this ultimate state being bliss – a not inappropriate image for the mysteries of creation, and one which goes some way toward explaining the origins of Tantrism. The Shri Yantra, used as a visual aid to help achieve one-pointedness of mind during meditation, is a diagram that illustrates just this concept. It starts from a single point, representing that of creation, surrounded by a pattern of interlocking triangles within layers of lotus petals, themselves set within a circle that symbolizes the cosmos. This circle opens out into a square whose sides act rather like mirrors reflecting in mirrors ad infinitum. The upward triangles represent the lingam and the downward ones, the yoni; their interpenetration the union of opposites, spirit and matter, male and female, creation and destruction, heaven and earth. As you gaze through these triangles to the space beyond, there is the point of infinity. Read from the inside out, the whole diagram represents the process of expanding creation, from the birth of consciousness to the outward manifestation of the material world. If you start from the outside and work inward, as a yogi meditating would do, you chart that process of withdrawal experienced by the meditator, away from the material world and toward a state of one-pointedness.

This use of art to express the mysteries of creation is not the sole preserve of yoga art. Most of us have heard of Zen art, and the sense of infinity and the layers of consciousness have been eloquently and beautifully expressed in the arts of Judaism, Christianity, and Islam throughout the ages. Modern and

Right. This familiar mandala, the Shri Yantra, not only represents the yogic vision of the cosmos, but is frequently used in meditation to draw the yogi inward.

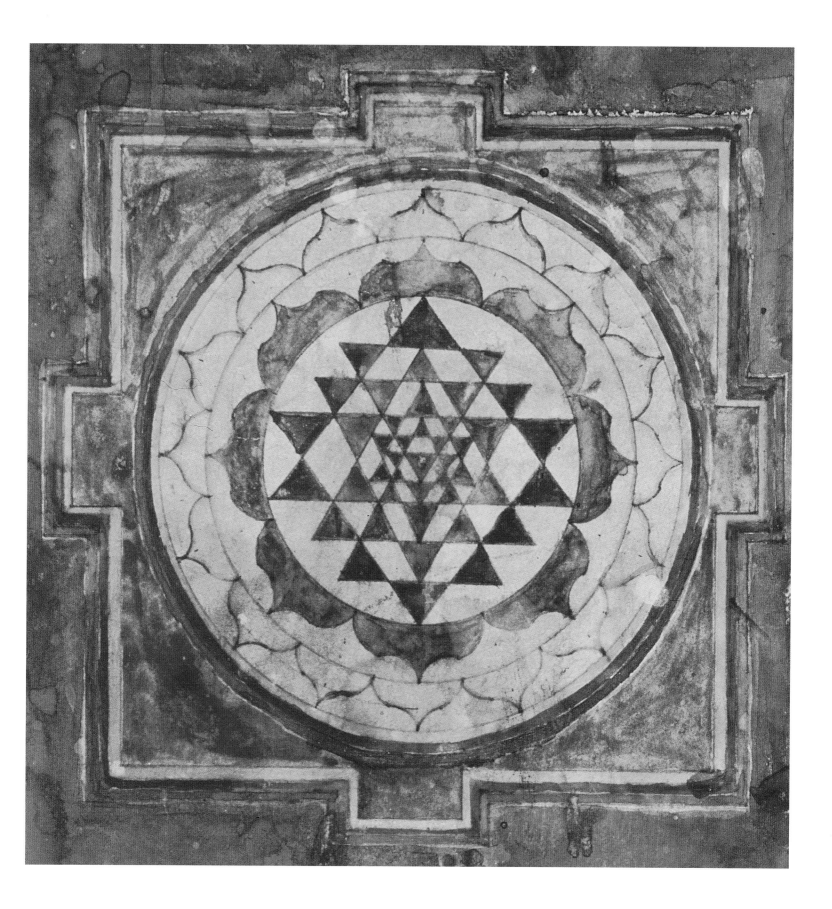

contemporary artists have worked on ideas more deliberately based on yoga. Brancusi, Klee, Kandinsky, Mondrian, and Rothko were all familiar with Theosophical interpretations of oriental philosophy. Kandinsky wrote: "The spiritual life to which art belongs, and of which it is one of the mightiest agents, is a complex but definite movement above and beyond, which can be translated into simplicity. The methods of the various arts are completely different externally. Sound, color, word. In their innermost core these methods are wholly identical. The final goal (knowledge) is reached through delicate vibrations of the human soul."

Patanjali explains how prakrti, or matter, itself is made up from a balance between three tendencies, known as the *gunas*. These gunas are *sattva*, which translates as clarity; *rajas*, activity; and *tamas*, inertia. These three principles are the basis of all matter, producing pleasure, pain, and indifference respectively. The theory is that that the interaction of these three gunas accounts for the ever-changing potential of experience. When the three elements are held in balance there is complete stillness. It is only when there is an imbalance of the equilibrium between them that the process of evolution can begin.

This page and overleaf. Every tradition, culture, and religion has explored the idea of "the One" as the source of all being. Modern and contemporary artists have expressed this sometimes with a conscious reference to yogic ideas.

Below left. A panel from a fifteenth-century inlaid wooden door. Each little piece is made separately and then fitted together in the Islamic starburst pattern, representing unity and infinity.

Below right. Illuminated manuscript depicting the Creation, from the Book of Hours, *painted in 1224 for a reading from the prophets for Holy Saturday.*

Right. White Dark III, *1995, by Anish Kapoor.*

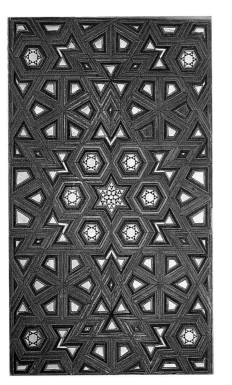

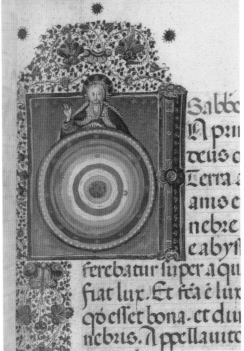

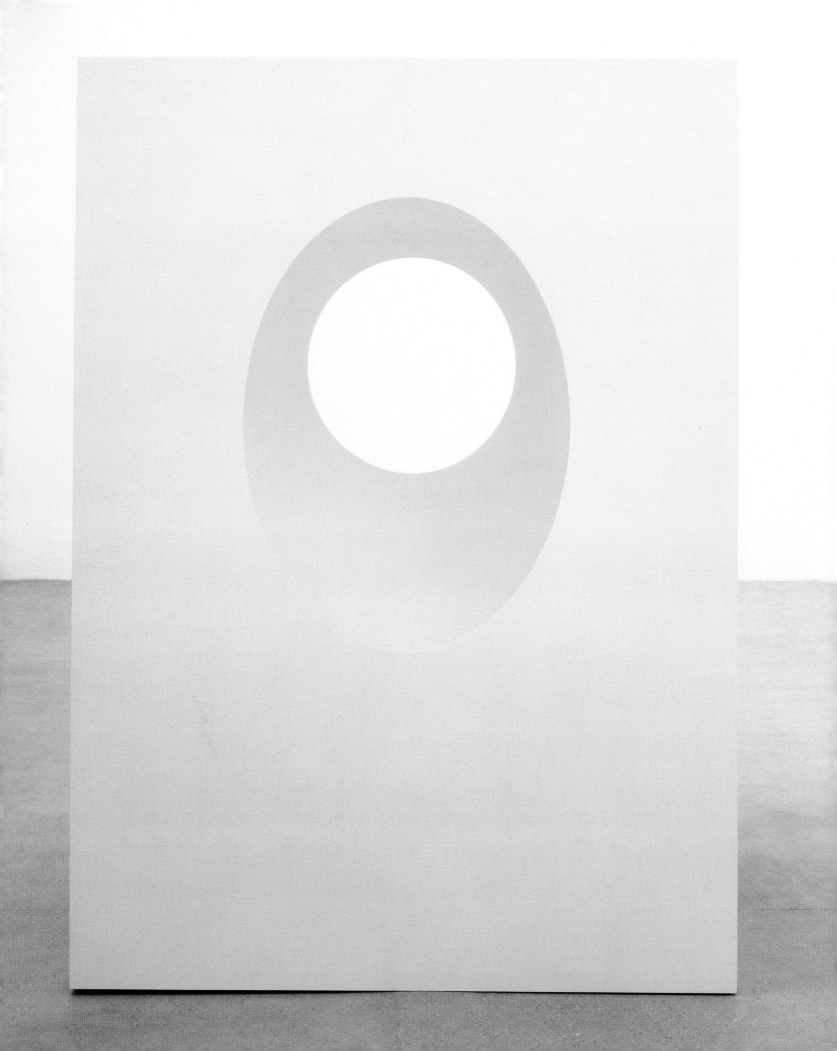

"See now the whole universe with all things that move and move not, and whatever thy soul may yearn to see. See it all as One in me." Krishna's exhortation to Arjuna in the Bhagavad Gita is appropriately illustrated by this diagram of the "Size of the Celestial Bodies" as estimated by the Dutchman Andrae Cellarius in 1661.

The void is not silent. I have always thought of it more and more as a transitional space, an in-between space... I have always been interested as an artist in how one can somehow look again for that very first moment of creativity where everything is possible and nothing has actually happened.

ANISH KAPOOR IN CONVERSATION
WITH H.K. BHABHA

The five obstacles to happiness listed by Patanjali are:

AVIDYA ~ *ignorance or wrong understanding, the root of all obstacles to happiness*

ASMITA ~ *egoism, the faulty identification of oneself with the instruments of the body and mind*

RAGA ~ *attachment, desiring something that has given you pleasure before*

DVESA ~ *aversion, fear of things that experience tells you can be unpleasant*

ABHINIVESA ~ *fear of death, the instinctive love of life and dread of death*

SINCE THE YOGA SYSTEM aims at the purification of the mind as a preparation for a spiritual enlightenment, Patanjali sets out in the Yoga Sutras the practical methods whereby the Self, the Atman personified in the *Bhagavad Gita* as Arjuna, can free itself from the afflictions of the ego in order to follow the path without distraction. "Experiences of pleasure and of pain are the fruits of merit and demerit respectively," says Patanjali in sutra fourteen of the second chapter, "But the man of spiritual discrimination regards all these experiences as painful. For even the enjoyment of present pleasure is painful, since we already fear its loss. Past pleasure is painful because renewed cravings arise from the impressions it has left upon the mind. And how can any happiness be lasting if it depends only upon our moods? For these moods are constantly changing, as one or another of the ever-warring gunas seizes control of the mind."

First we must differentiate between the Self and the ego, because the conscious Self is essentially pure while the ego, dependent on one's personal experience of the world, inevitably distorts that experience. Suffering is said to be caused by ignorance of the true nature of the world, *avidya*. Self is separate from matter, and to understand this distinction is to release oneself from suffering. Patanjali explains this misguided identification of the Atman with the ego, and lists the five causes of such misguidedness, which become obstacles to happiness and create all suffering (see left). Put another way, self-interest, self-gratification, vanity, and self-delusion can never be the route to peace and happiness, to morality, or to the foundation of any religious discipline.

The special feature of the yoga system is the practical set of rules it lays down, which, if followed, will lead the yogi "to advance toward the light": "As soon as all impurities have been removed by the practice of the limbs of yoga, a man's spiritual vision opens to the light-giving knowledge of the Atman," says Patanjali. These eight limbs include a moral code for behavior toward oneself and the world around one, postures, breathing, and meditation. Patanjali called them the path of Ashtanga Yoga, the eightfold path. Some people define this as the path of Raja Yoga. These eight principles are a guide toward perfect yoga, which is the route to union with the universal spirit, or purusha; by following this path the yogi can ultimately attain a wider and deeper knowledge of the dimensions of life, can transcend reality and find bliss. The eight steps of Patanjali's system are:

YAMA

abstention

NIYAMA

observance

ASANA

posture

PRANAYAMA

breath control

PRATYAHARA

withdrawal of the senses

DHARANA

fixed attention

DHYANA

contemplation

SAMADHI

concentration

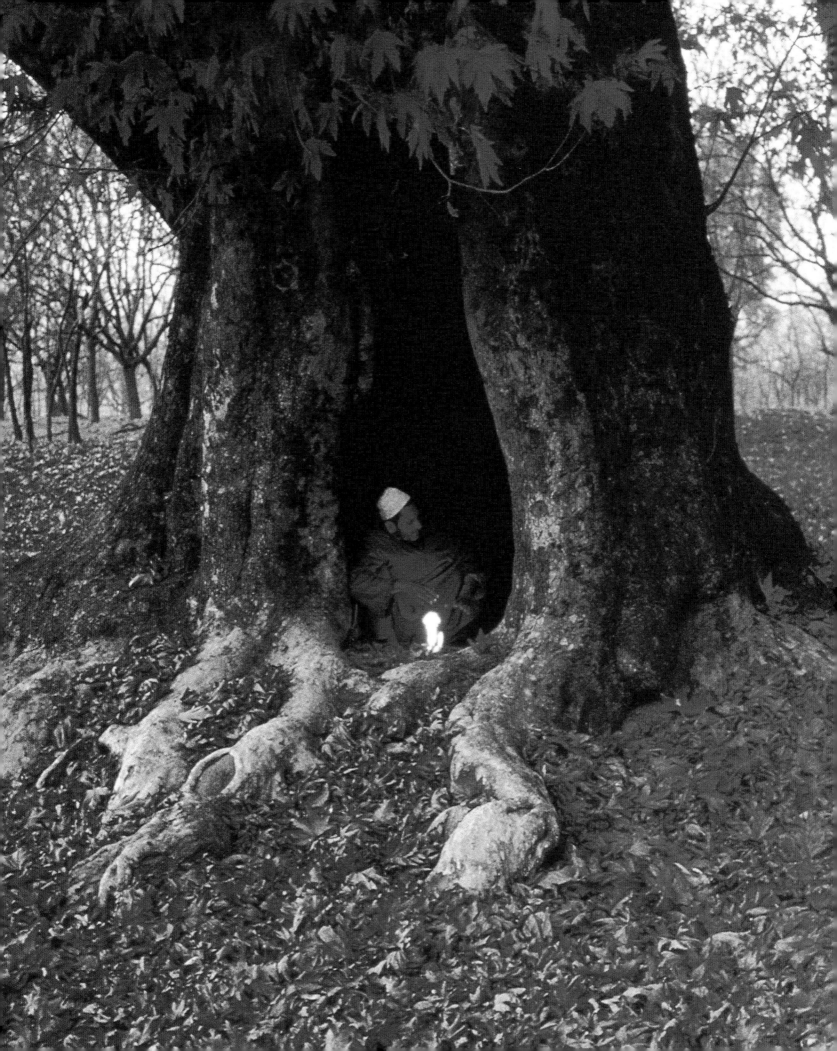

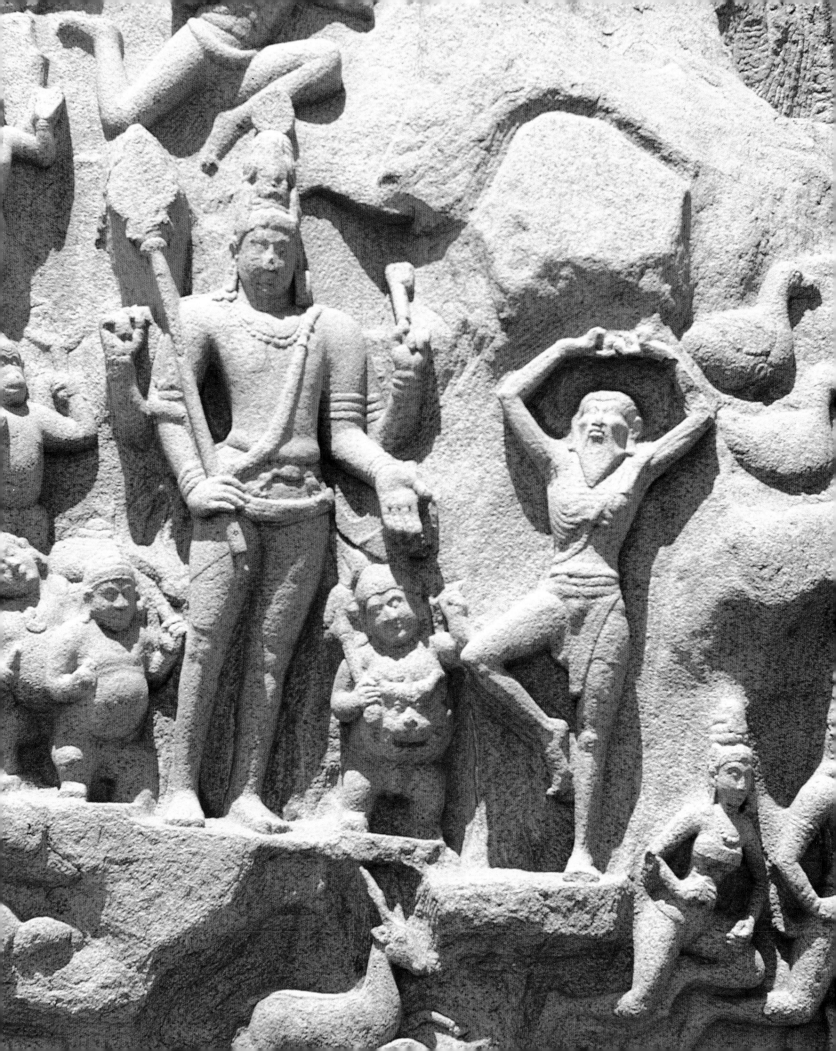

Left. "Perfection of the body includes beauty, grace, strength, and adamantine hardness," says Patanjali. This temple carving of Arjuna standing in a position suspiciously like Tree pose is in Mahabali Pooram.

YAMA ~ The first step to enlightenment must be to deal with the world around you in a moral way. The five prescriptions that make up yama have much in common with the moral commandments of Buddhist and Jain practices. The first is *ahimsa*, which means nonviolence and can be interpreted as living without harming others in thought, word, or deed. *Satya* demands truthfulness, and on the subject of *asteya,* which is not to steal, sutra thirty-seven says, tantalizingly: "When a man becomes steadfast in his abstention from theft, all wealth comes to him." *Brahmacharya* is chastity or celibacy, suggesting that one on the path of yoga would refrain from sex so as to be free from attachment and from its diverting influence. A more contemporary interpretation might be that sex should not be squandered lustfully. The fifth and last yama is *aparigraha*, which is interpreted as abstaining from greed. Not being acquisitive is clearly an essential quality for one who is striving for nonattachment. Aparigraha also covers the receiving of gifts that could be considered as bribes.

NIYAMA ~ In order to be in a fit state for concentration on higher things, the body, too, must be purified. "Cleanliness is next to Godliness" says the Christian Church, and the yogi applies these principles by beginning with a pure diet, *sauca*, and simple physical hygiene to bring him closer to God. He must also have a clean or unperverted mind, according to Patanjali. The unclean mind is interpreted in Christopher Isherwood's and Swami Prabhavananda's commentary on of the Yoga Sutras as one in danger of lack of discrimination: "The danger in gossip, light entertainment, ephemeral journalism, popular fiction, radio romancing, etc, is simply this. They encourage us to drift into a relaxed reverie, neutral at first but soon colored by anxieties, addictions, and aversions so that the mind becomes dark and impure."

The second niyama, *samtosa*, is concerned with contentment. The yogi must accept and face reality without emotion. Fame or anonymity, pleasure or pain, gain or loss, success or failure are all the same. *Tapas* is the third niyama, which translates as austerity. This introduces the element of ascetism to the path of yoga, thought to be necessary if the yogi is to prove he is dependent on nothing. The Russian devotional classic, *The Way of the Pilgrim*, tells of a life of tapas, and many of the most celebrated gurus and sages have spent years alone in meditation with the bare necessities of life on their personal path to yoga. Like the *Bhagavad Gita*, Patanjali is clear, however, that tapas is about self-control and not about the obsessive or even masochistic extremes to which some are inclined to take asceticism. *Svadhyaya*, the fourth niyama, points to the benefits of continuous learning and study, while the fifth, *ishvarapranidhana*, requires that all actions be carried out through devotion to God. This is another form of nonattachment – that one does not fall into the trap of doing something for the sake of the fruits of that action but for the sake of the action itself and for love of God.

ASANA ~ Asana is the practice of postures to bring about a strong and sound body, which can in turn contribute to a balanced approach to training the mind. Asanas give the body a sense of grounding, which in turn leads to a release of energy.

After mastering posture, one must practice control of the prana by stopping the motions of inhalation and exhalation.
PATANJALI

When the five senses and the mind are still, and reason itself rests in silence, then begins the Path supreme. This calm steadiness is called Yoga. Then one should become watchful, because Yoga comes and goes.
KATHA UPANISHAD

When in meditation, the true nature of the object shines forth, not distorted by the mind of the perceiver, that is samadhi.
PATANJALI

PRANAYAMA ~ This is the only place in the Yoga Sutras where Patanjali stipulates that one must not attempt one of the eight limbs until another has been mastered – implying much about the power of the breath. Pranayama is a physical means to a spiritual end. Because of the close relationship between the flow of the breath and a person's mental state, balanced breathing can promote mental equilibrium and clarity. However, over-indulgence in breathing exercises may lead to hallucinations and possibly even insanity.

PRATYAHARA ~ This is the first purely mental step in Patanjali's eightfold path. Pratyahara translates as withdrawal of the mind from sense objects. The mind is made clear by right breathing, the body is healthy and pure, and it is at this point that attention can be withdrawn from external objects and distractions.

DHARANA ~ Dharana is pure concentration, sustained to bring about *ekagrata*, or one-pointedness of the mind, so that it can focus exclusively and unwaveringly on one thing. This is usually achieved through the use of a mantra, mandala, or some other tool that can help the mind find its focus. Many of the prerequisites for meditation given in the yogic texts are here in the *Philokalia*, one of the great works of Christian mysticism: "Sit down alone and in silence. Lower your head, shut your eyes, breathe out gently, and imagine yourself looking into your own heart. As you breathe out, say, 'Lord Jesus Christ, have mercy on me.' Say it moving your lips gently, or simply say it in your mind. Try to put all other thoughts aside. Be calm, be patient, and repeat the process very frequently. Collect your mind, lead it into the path of the breath along which the air enters in, constrain it to enter the heart altogether with inhaled air, and keep it there."

DHYANA ~ This is meditation or contemplation. Pure dhyana is reached when dharana becomes spontaneous and unbroken. The process of meditation has been compared to the pouring of oil from one vessel into another in a steady stream. The thought waves in the mind calm into one perfect continuity of thought, and once this has been mastered it leads to samadhi, the last of the eight limbs of yoga.

SAMADHI ~ This is the transcendental state that is the end of all yoga practice. The last three stages of the eightfold path are linked together. Patanjali states that it is no use to attempt meditation without mastering concentration, and without these first two it is not possible to progress to samadhi, which is the ultimate aim of the yogi's quest and a liberation from reality into a subtle and highly spiritual experience.

The warning in the *Katha Upanishad*, that "yoga comes and goes" is one that crops up in other texts time and again. Patanjali's system for reaching enlightenment is in itself an acknowledgment that even if enlightenment has been achieved, once the work is abandoned, enlightenment will slip away.

Right. Shiva is depicted in many incarnations – as the awe-inspiring god of destruction, performing his dance of creation to time's rhythm, and here in the altogether more gentle guise of the Great Yogi.

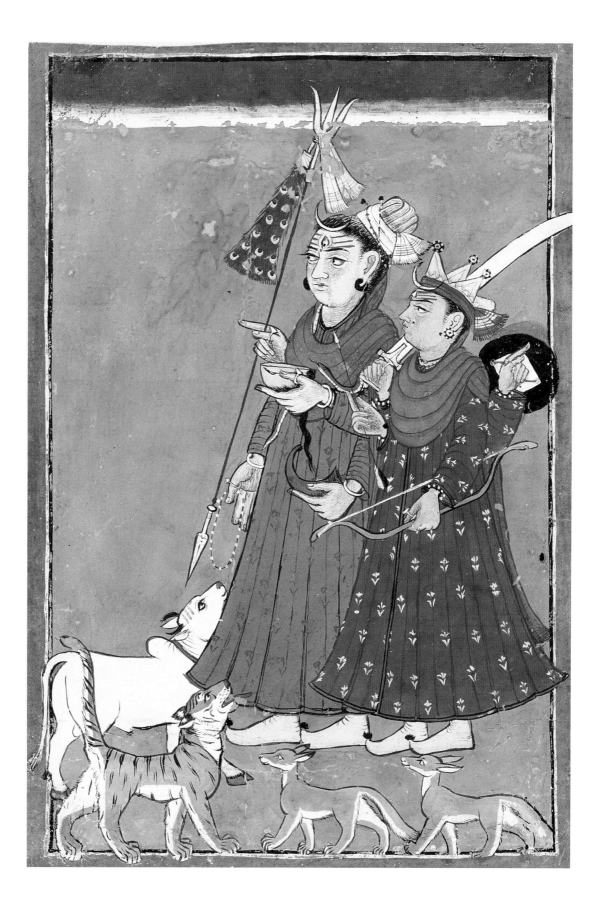

When thy mind leaves behind its dark forests of delusion, thou shalt go beyond the scriptures of times past and still to come.

BHAGAVAD GITA

THE SCHOLAR PERIOD ~ In a sense we are still in the so-called scholar period, in that the scriptures and sutras are all still being analyzed, interpreted, and commented on. While Patanjali's system may be the one for the purists, it is not the only source of inspiration for the many paths of yoga that developed in his wake. The Western mind has become fascinated by Indian writings more than ever before, and particularly by the Indian focus on the spiritual aspect of life. In Indian philosophy, material welfare is not considered to be the goal of human life, and philosophy and religion are intimately related. There has always been a close relationship between theory and practice, between the belief system and life as it is lived.

YOGA PATHS

HATHA YOGA ~ It is said that all forms of yoga begin with Hatha and end with Raja. Most yoga practitioners in the West practice Hatha Yoga in some form or other, and the general understanding of this has been that Hatha Yoga is concerned with the practice of asanas, or postures, for the purpose of balancing, purifying and strengthening the body, and Raja Yoga with the meditative aspect. It is true that the Hatha Yoga texts put their emphasis on the physical aspects of yoga practice. Nevertheless, Hatha Yoga contains all the elements of Patanjali's eight limbs of classical yoga, so the modern distinction between the two is a misinterpretation. The *Hatha Yoga Pradipika* explains that the aim of Hatha Yoga is to unify the energies of HA (the sun, the male principle and the right side) with THA (the moon, the female principle and the left side), merging them into the energy channel, the *susumna*, in the center of the spine. One of the translations of the word yoga is union. To understand this one must explore the concept of kundalini, one that lies at the heart of all types of yoga, not just Tantric philosophy.

KUNDALINI YOGA ~ The principle of kundalini comes from that of the subtle body. This is not something you can cut open the body and pinpoint, and the actual meaning and interpretation of kundalini and its awakening, or raising, is surrounded by a lot of mystery and superstition. But if you equate the power of kundalini to that of prana, or vital energy, it is more easily understood. Vital energy is said to be so fine that it makes some layers of the body undetectable by modern scientific investigation. At this level there is an inner universe permeated by prana, and this life-force is channeled along pathways known as *nadis*. There are hundreds of nadis, but two

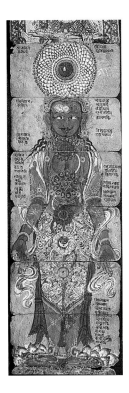

A late nineteenth-century representation of the chakras, from Rajasthan, showing the full flowering of the kundalini principle above the head.

of the principal ones are the *pingala*, which carries the solar energy, HA, and the *ida*, which carries the lunar energy, THA. Yoga aims to channel the prana into the central channel, the susumna nadi, which lies along the axis of the spine – as do the channels of the nervous system. The hot energy of the sun and the cool energy of the moon twist around the spine, meeting it at six points. These are the six chakras.

At the base of the six points and blocking the susumna channel is the dormant energy, symbolized by a coiled serpent, representing the female energy of prakrti, and known as the kundalini. The aim of some Hatha and Tantric practices is to arouse this dormant energy, this serpent, and drive it up the susumna nadi, activating the chakras along the way until they all unite in the final, seventh, chakra, the seat of the male energy, the purusha, at the crown of the head. This results in transformation. You could also call it truth, bliss, nirvana, heaven, awakening, or enlightenment. It is not like a thunderbolt, an electric shock, or even an incredible orgasm – as intriguing imagery of the Serpent Goddess and the lotus centers of energy occasionally suggest – and it is misleading, and in some cases dangerous, that it is referred to in this way. When you sit in meditation regularly and the distractions of a scattered mind are calm and uncluttered, it is possible to glimpse and sense a rebalancing and a release of energy. Then it becomes clear that all the paths or directions of yoga are dealing with the same thing, to calm the mind and lead us to the same ultimate union or yoga.

TANTRIC YOGA ~ No one knows how old Tantrism is. The earliest surviving texts are Buddhist and date to about 600 C.E., but there are many elements of what became Tantra in much more ancient scriptures from both Hindu and Buddhist traditions. In Nepal, Buddhist and Hindu Tantra merged, and Hindu Tantra was adopted in Southeast Asia. It was assimilated and occasionally combined with Muslim ideas and traveled to many other countries, including China and Japan. It flourished in Tibet from the seventh century, and Tibetan Tantra went to Mongolia. No wonder its interpretations are various and often misleading.

Tantra translates as technique, implying a skill or craft. In the Tantric texts there is emphasis on secrecy and on the importance of initiation by a guru. The texts themselves take the form of dialogues between the god Shiva and his female counterpart, Durga, or Shakti. They are epic poems and coded writings full of symbolism and ritual, jungles and snakes, female deities and orgies, phallic cults and magic practices. The religious systems' traditional to orthodox Brahmins argue that the real world is utterly without value and that we must pry ourselves away from the things we care about most, such as love for our lover, children, food, music, art, and possessions, because they are traps. We learn techniques of abstinence and meditation in order to attain detachment from these worthless distractions. The Tantric idea is in complete contrast to this. It asserts that instead of suppressing pleasure, vision, and ecstasy, these should be cultivated and used for good; that it is by using the body as a vehicle that one can reach enlightenment. This is not a free rein for indulgence in animal passions for the sake of sheer pleasure. Hindu Tantrism claims that everything, bad and good, is the action of the female creative principle. Shakti is generally represented in a carnal embrace with Shiva, the god who generated her for his own enjoyment. Of course they are ultimately one person, a double-sexed deity involved in blissful intercourse with itself. At a superficial level this can be interpreted as an exercise in raising the human libido, and indeed this is a frequent interpretation of raising the kundalini, but at a deeper level

Tantrism, like yoga, sees the human body as a reflection of the cosmos and vice versa. The two are, so to speak, the same system, and one is inconceivable without the other. The Tantrika does cultivate methods aimed at arousing dormant energies, but once aroused through ritual meditation and yoga, the energy is turned inward and used to propel the practitioner toward enlightenment. Tantrism is not a faith, but a way of life, distinct from, but not incompatible with, traditional ways, which is how it has found its way into so many traditions.

The faithful of the cult of Tantra regarded sexual intercourse as an essential rite of initiation, enabling them to attain knowledge. The male and female principles merge in the couple and transcend the sexual embrace.

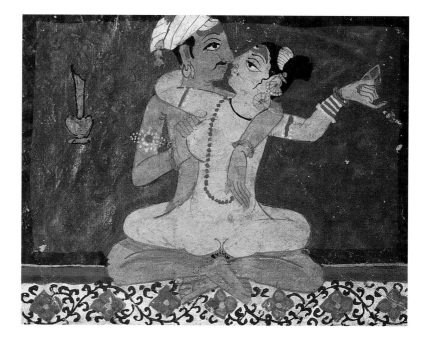

RAJA YOGA ~ *Raja* means king in Sanskrit. In the context of Raja Yoga the word is used metaphorically — when one reaches enlightenment one becomes a king among men. One interpretation of Raja Yoga links it with the concept of *isvara*, or God. In other words, finding God. The word isvara is sometimes even interchanged with the word raja in the Vedas. Alternatively, you can think of raja as the king within each of us. This potential for greatness is hidden by everyday distractions, fantasies, and sensuality. But with practice, the mind can take control of the senses and by reaching that level we can find clarity and peace. Traditionally, Raja Yoga is associated with the classical yoga system of Patanjali. Today there exist groups that have taken the name Raja Yoga to endorse what is actually just another religious sect. These have little to do with the sort of yoga we have been talking about.

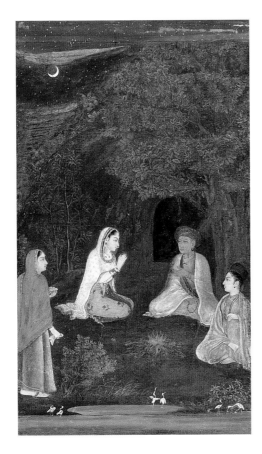

This eighteenth-century painting of a lady visiting an ashram at night seems to indicate that yoga and the spiritual path was never the exclusive preserve of men.

JNANA YOGA ~ Jnana Yoga describes the aspect of yoga that concerns the search for real knowledge. It is the intellectual approach to spiritual evolution through inquiry and constant self-analysis. The underlying hypothesis of Jnana Yoga is that all knowledge is hidden within us, we only have to access it. Traditionally the search for this hidden knowledge starts with it being passed down from teacher to student and through interpretations of the ancient scriptures. After discussion and reflection there is a gradual recognition of the truth and a merging with it. The state of true understanding is samadhi.

BHAKTI YOGA ~ *Bhakti* comes from the root *bhaj*, to serve. This is not about service to a person but to a power greater than ourselves. Bhakti Yoga concerns the devotional side of yoga, the recognition of God as truth. This could be described as the mystical path of yoga, in which God is served, unquestioningly, at all times, through meditating on and speaking his name, and living with him at all times.

KRIYA YOGA ~ There are different ideas about the definition of Kriya Yoga. According to the sutras, the whole spectrum of practices known as yoga could be called Kriya Yoga. However, there are three aspects that are important in Kriya Yoga, and they are tapas, svadhyaya, and isvarapranidhana. We have encountered all three of these in Patanjali's niyamas. Tapas is associated with practices, like asanas and pranayama, that can help us to remove blocks or afflictions, both physical and mental, through discipline. Svadhyaya is the asking of questions and self-examination, and isvarapranidhana is the carrying out of actions that are not motivated by outcome. All of these three elements touch on every other aspect of yoga already discussed, but these particular three taken together have a joint concern with purification that defines them as Kriya Yoga. Kriya Yoga should not be confused with the kriyas, the cleansing techniques that were described in part two.

KARMA YOGA ~ Karma is a Sanskrit word much overused and abused by people who don't understand it. The word *karma* means action, or work, and the consequences of action. Krishna explains to Arjuna in the *Bhagavad Gita* that in life we can only act, but that our actions should never be affected by expectations we might have of them or their perceived successes or failures. The law of karma is the law of universal cause and effect that binds man with the universe. It is this law that decides what are the effects of our actions; our perception of whether they've been a success or a failure is irrelevant and amounts to nothing more than pure distraction. Karma Yoga, then, is the yoga of selfless action.

Ascetics have long held a fascination for princes and emperors, whose visits to these hermits for sage advice – their realities so different from the life of pomp and circumstance at court – are a common subject of illustrations.

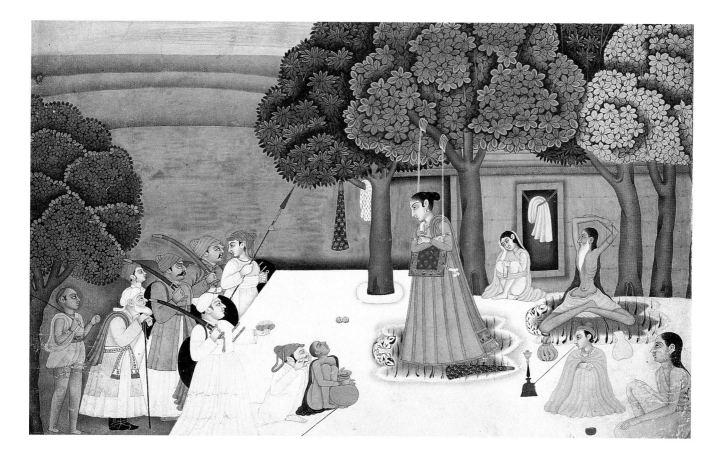

I'm not here to tell you how this is going to end. I'm here to tell you how it's going to begin.

NEO, PLAYED BY KEANU REEVES IN *THE MATRIX*

IF YOGIS AND ASCETICS have long been sought out by kings and princes for their advice, one early western traveler to India, a seventeenth-century French gem trader by the name of Tavernier, doubted the authenticity of many of the faquirs he came across, using familiar language: "They are all of them vagabonds and lazy drones that dazzle the eyes of the people with a false zeal, and make them believe that whatever comes out of their mouths is an oracle." Nevertheless, he observed one sadhu locking himself in a hut without food or drink for days on end as, "a thing which I could not have believed had I not seen it. The president of the Dutch Company set a spy to watch night and day, whether anybody brought him any victuals. But he could not discover any relief the faquir had, all the while sitting upon his bum like our tailors, never changing his posture above seven days together."

By the time of British rule in India, many commentators, both native and British, had found that the standards of Hindu practice and scholarship had slipped. One great early nineteenth-century reformer, Ram Mohan, a Brahmin living in Calcutta, said that Hinduism had degenerated because its uneducated masses were not familiar with the true spirit of their faith as expressed in the Vedas and Upanishads. This, he believed, had made them vulnerable to the machinations of unscrupulous and self-seeking priests who played on their superstitions and fears. These priests, together with what the scholar Julius Lipner describes as "rampant polytheism, idolatry and ritualism, which was riddled with the canker of priestcraft and such abominable social practices as suttee, and caste and sex discrimination," had brought Hinduism into disrepute. Ram Mohan was convinced that the remedy for this was to go back to the Upanishads. He became one of the key figures in the movement for Hindu reform, preparing it, perhaps, for the burst of Western enthusiasm and interest that was to appear from the mid-nineteenth century onward.

The uniqueness of yoga, according to some philosophers, is that it is based on a living tradition and yet has translated to a popular level to be studied and applied by an incredibly wide audience, and not necessarily one with a similar cultural background. Although Jung felt that yoga could never be assimilated in the West, it seems he was wrong. Its appeal has increased rather than diminished, particularly when compared to that of other ancient mystical traditions such as, say, Greek mysteries, Ancient Egyptian magic, forms of shamanism or medieval Christian mysticism. However, to the purist, the form that yoga takes in the West today is an easy path in comparison to the ritualistic and ascetic outlook of the yogis of the Brahmanic culture. For the latter, the path of the true yogi is that of renouncing all material and worldly cares, obligations and aims, and concentrating on the search for final truth. Many wandering ascetics led long lives devoted to yoga that involved not only years of study with a teacher but later a time of enforced poverty and homelessness, when the yogi spent his existence as a hermit, working and praying and wandering the country without attachments, making sure that when death came, he left no trace of himself whatsoever.

These traditional garlands evoke the richness of color and the exoticism associated with India.

"Through pleasure and pain, through good and evil, the infinite river of souls is flowing into the ocean of perfection, of self-realization."

SWAMI VIVEKANANDA

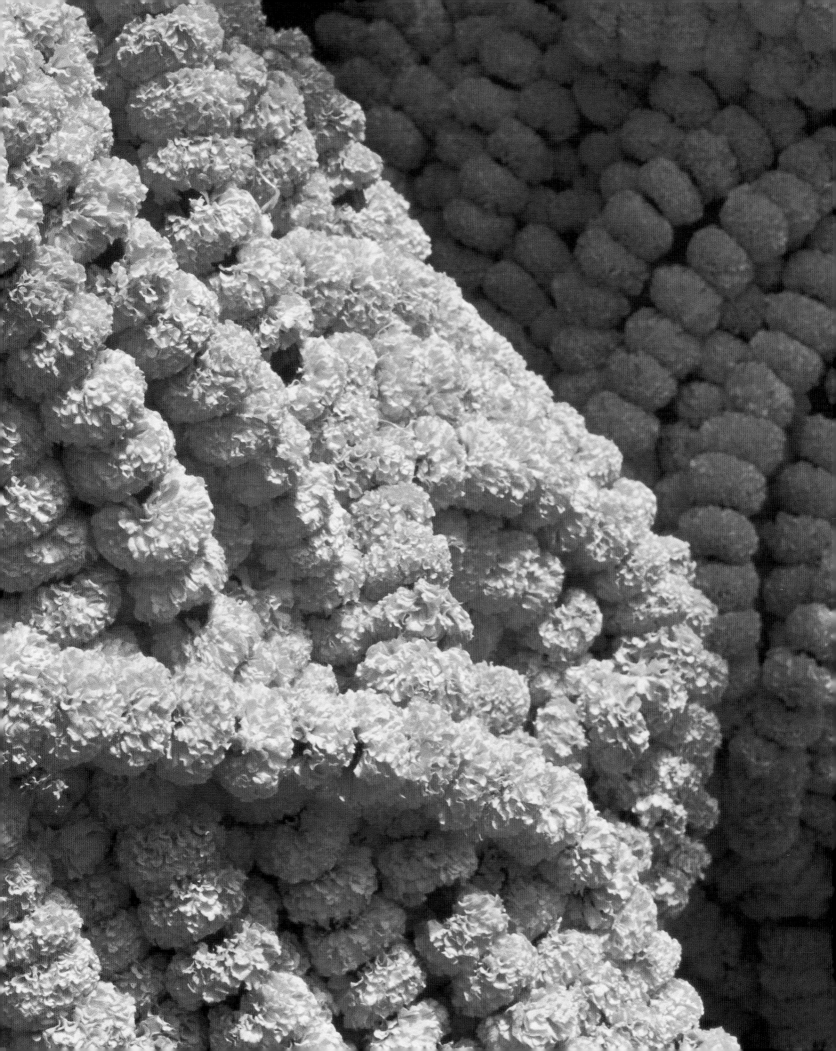

GLOSSARY OF SANSKRIT TERMS

ABHINIVESA ~ *fear (see also avidya).*

AHIMSA ~ *nonviolence.*

ASMITA ~ *ego (see also avidya).*

ATMAN ~ *immortal soul, the Self.*

AUM ~ *the single infinite sound from which all the elements and gunas originated; in other words, the sound of the creation of the universe. A sacred sound that is often used in meditation. Also written as* OM.

AVIDYA ~ *variously translated as incorrect understanding, misapprehension, or ignorance – what comes between a person and his or her ability to fulfill the true state of yoga. The most important of a total of five obstacles, the others being asmita, raga, dvesa, and abhinivesa.*

BHAKTI ~ *devotion. Bhakti Yoga emphasises devotion or love.*

DARSANA ~ *literally, a way of seeing, more specifically seeing inside. It has come to refer to the six classical systems of view of Indian thought. Patanjali systemized yoga as a darsana in its own right (alongside Vedanta, Mimamsa, Samkhya, Vaisesika, and Nyaya). Also defined as the science of knowledge or philosophy.*

DVESA ~ *refusal (see also avidya).*

GUNA ~ *quality or tendency. There are three gunas: rajas, sattva, and tamas, and between them they define the state of the universe, as well as being qualities of mind.*

JNANA ~ *knowledge. Jnana Yoga is the form of yoga that emphasises inquiry and analysis.*

KAIVALYA ~ *final emancipation; the liberation of purusha; the ultimate state of yoga – freedom.*

KARMA ~ *action or work, both mental and physical, and the rule that makes these affect the future. The concept of karma is, therefore, closely bound up with that of reincarnation and the cycle of rebirth from*

which Hindus and Buddhists are trying to free themselves.

MAYA ~ *illusion, specifically the physical world of apparent multiplicity that blinds us to the reality – unity – behind it. Maya is also the power in nature that creates this illusion.*

MOKSHA ~ *final emancipation, liberation.*

OM ~ *see* AUM.

PRAKRTI ~ *matter, the primitive, non-intelligent principle, also the female energy, composed of the three gunas. When it embraces purusha, the two become a single principle, experienced as the transcendence of duality. The concept of prakrti explains why true insight cannot come from human intellect, because the intellect is itself a part of prakrti.*

PURUSHA ~ *Life force, vital energy, the breath.*

PURUSHA ~ *spirit, pure consciousness. The primeval male / inert spirit that conjoins with prakrti to produce the universe. It is purusha that becomes clouded by avidya.*

RAJA ~ *Raja Yoga is defined variously as "The path of psychic control… suitable for a man of mystic temperament" (Swami Sivananda) and "Yoga in which union with the highest power is the goal" (T. K. V. Desikachar). Often it refers to the yoga of Patanjali.*

RAJAS ~ *one of the gunas. This is the quality of activity, dust, and passion. It is on the same wavelength as the color red, is the sound* A *in* AUM, *and is represented by a semicircle.*

RTA ~ *unalloyed truth, as opposed to truths that make conceptual sense but that describe only notions of the analytical mind.*

SADHANA ~ *practice.*

SAMSKARA ~ *a state that is latent in the subconscious mind that predisposes*

someone to a certain pattern of behavior, which can be mental or physical. It can lead to avidya.

SATTVA ~ *another one of the gunas, sattva is the quality of clarity and lightness and stands for the cosmic intellect. Its color is white, its sound is the* U *of* AUM, *and it is represented by the straight line.*

SRUTI ~ *the Vedas, or words, of the sages.*

SUTRA ~ *literally "thread." Also, that which runs through and holds things together, hence aphorisms, treatises, and the Yoga Sutras of Patanjali. Also implicit in this meaning is the linking of teacher, teaching, and student.*

TAMAS ~ *this guna is the quality of heaviness, darkness, inertia, and stability. Its tendency is toward disintegration, its color black, its sound the* M *of* AUM, *and it is represented by a point.*

TAPAS ~ *asceticism. Also translated as the controlling of physical appetites and passions, purification, and self-discipline, mental, moral, and physical.*

YAMA ~ *universal moral commandment.*

YOGI or YOGIN ~ *male practitioner of yoga.*

YOGINI ~ *female practitioner of yoga.*

FURTHER READING

ANATOMY

Calais-Germain, Blandine
~ *Anatomy of Movement*, 1993

Todd, Mabel Elsworth
~ *The Thinking Body*, 1937

YOGA IN PRACTICE

Desikachar, T.K.V., and R.H. Cravens
~ *Health, Healing and Beyond;
Yoga and the Living Tradition of
Krishnamacharya*, 1998

Desikachar, T.K.V.
~ *The Heart of Yoga*, 1995

Farhi, Donna
~ *The Breathing Book: Good Health
and Vitality Through Essential Breath
Work,* 1996

Freemantle, Chloë
~ *Yoga Practise Handbook*, 2000

Iyengar, B.K.S.
~ *Light on Yoga*, revised edition, 2001

Myers, Esther
~ *Yoga and You*, 1996

Sabatini, Sandra
~ *Breath, the Essence of Yoga*, 2000

Scaravelli, Vanda
~ *Awakening the Spine*, 1991

Schiffman, Erich
~ *Yoga: The Spirit and Practice of
Moving into Stillness*, 1996

Stewart, Mary
~ *Yoga Over 50*, 1994

Stewart, Mary
~ *Teach Yourself Yoga*, 1998

Stewart, Mary, and Kathy Phillips
~ *Yoga for Children*, 1992

INDIAN PHILOSOPHY, LITERATURE, AND ART

Craven, Roy
~ *A Concise History of Indian Art*, 1976

Easwaran, Eknath (tr.)
~ *The Upanishads*, 1987

Eliade, Mircea
~ *Yoga, Immortality and Freedom*, 1990

Hariharananda Aranya, tr. P.N. Mukerji
~ *Yoga Philosophy of Patanjali*, 1983

Khanna, Balraj, and George Michell
~ *Human and Divine; 2000 Years of
Indian Sculpture*, 2000

Lipner, Julius
~ *Hindus, their Religious Beliefs and
Practices*, 1994

Mascaro, Juan (tr.)
~ *Bhagavad Gita*, 1962

Mascaro, Juan (tr.)
~ *The Upanishads*, 1965

Mookherjee, Ajit
~ *Yoga Art*, 1975

Muktananda
~ *Secret of the Siddhas*, 1980

Prabhavananada and Christopher
Isherwood
~ *How to Know God: The Yoga
Aphorisms of Patanjali*, 1981

Radhakrishnan, Sarvepalli, and
Charles Moore
~ *Sourcebook of Indian Philosophy*,
1989

Radice, Betty (ed.)
~ *Hindu Myths*, 1975

Rawson, Philip
~ *The Art of Tantra*, 1973

Warner, Karel
~ *Yoga and Indian Philosophy*, 1989

MYSTICISM AND SPIRITUALISM IN OTHER TRADITIONS

Chopra, Deepak
~ *How to Know God*, 2000

Goldsmith, Joel S.
~ *Conscious Union with God*, 1993

His Holiness the Dalai Lama
~ *The Good Heart*, 1996

Khalil Gibran, ed. Robin Waterfield
~ *The Voice of Khalil Gibran*, 1995

Main, John
~ *Word into Silence*, 1980

Main, John
~ *The Way of Unknowing*, 1989

Schimmel, Annemarie
~ *Mystical Dimensions of Islam*, 1975

Revel, Jean-François, and Matthieu Ricard
~ *The Monk and the Philosopher;
East Meets West in a Father–Son
Dialogue*, 1998

Rumi, Jalaleddin, tr. Coleman Barks with
John Moyne
~ *Whoever Brought Me Here Will Have
to Take Me Home*, 1995

Washington, Peter
~ *Madame Blavatsky's Baboon*, 1995

Wolters, Clifton (tr.)
~ *The Cloud of Unknowing*, 1978

INDIA, NEPAL, AND TIBET

Archer, William and Mildred
~ *India Served and Observed*, 1994

Dowman, Keith
~ *The Power Places of Kathmandu*, 1995

Jack, Ian (ed.)
~ *India, Granta vol. 57*, 1997

Maraini, Fosco
~ *Secret Tibet*, 2000

Mehta, Gita
~ *Karma Cola*, 1979

NOVELS

Hesse, Herman, tr. Hilda Rosner
~ *Siddhartha*, 1954

Pirsig, Robert M.
~ *Zen and the Art of Motorcycle
Maintenance*, 1974

Seth, Vikram
~ *A Suitable Boy*, 1993

OTHER

Harris, Judith
~ *Jung and Yoga*, 2000

Jung, C.G.
~ *Psychology and the East*, 1986

Jung, C.G.
~ *Man and His Symbols*, 1964

Reid, Daniel P.
~ *The Tao of Health, Sex and
Longevity*, 1989

INDEX

addiction 56
Adho Mukha Svanasana 86–87
aerobics 24, 48, 67
ailments 56–57
Alexander Technique, The 60
Anthroposophy 32
Ardha Chandrasana 80–81
Ardha Matsyendrasana 104–105
asanas 64–121, 172, 175
ascetics 186
Ashtanga Yoga 37, 48–49, 172
AUM 134, 149
Avidya 170, 171
Ayurvedic medicine 43–44, 54

backache 56
Backbend from Standing 82–83
Baddha Konasana 112–113
Bakasana 94–95
Bandhas 126
Beatles, The 20, 42, 43
Besant, Annie 31, 32
Bhagavad Gita 37, 54, 149–151,
    152–156, 171, 173
Bhakti Yoga 37, 182
Bhujangasana 96–97
bibliography 189
Bikram Yoga 47–48
Blavatsky, Helena 29–32, 34
body postures 65
Bound Angle 112–113
Bow 98–99
Brahmins 163, 186
Bramari 129
breathing
    art of 128–129
    awareness 67
    controlled 65, 122–129
    correct 68
    diaphragm 68, 128
    exercises 129
Buddhism 139, 141, 156, 159,
    160–161
Busia, Kofi 10

celebrities 15, 18–20, 49
Chataranga Dandasana 86
Chidvilasananda, Gurumayi 33, 40
Child's pose 57, 110–111

China 58–60, 84
Chopra, Deepak 33
cleansing processes 126
Cobblers 57, 112–113
Cobra 9, 23, 96–97
Cobra unwinds 60
Concentration 131
constipation 56
contemplation 154
Corpse 57, 71, 120–121
Cow 57
Crane 94–95

Dao-yin 59, 67
depression 56
Desikachar, T.K.V. 44, 47, 54, 132
Dharana 131, 132, 134, 172, 176
Dhyana 131, 134, 172, 176
diaphragm 68, 128
diet 54–55
Dog 57, 86–87

Eagle 22–23, 57, 60
ego and Self, difference 171
eightfold path 171–176
Eka Pada Rajakapotasana 100–101, 103
Eliade, Mircea 123
epic writings 150–157
eye strain 56

feet 84–85
Feldenkrais 26, 61
Forward Bend 56, 57, 100,
    106–107, 118
Full Prostration 118

Ganges, River 17, 18
gravity 68
Great Yogi 177
Guruji *see* B.K.S. Iyengar
gurus today 33–34

Half Moon 80–81
"Hatha Fusion" 49
Hatha Yoga 37, 40, 115, 162, 180
headache 57
Headstand 10, 11, 47, 57, 88,
    92–93, 95
Headstand Backarch 95

health promoted by yoga 51–52, 56–57
Healthy Happy Holy Foundation 48
Himalaya mountains 139
Hinduism 139, 141, 159, 186
hip stiffness 57
historical chart 38–39

Illumination 131
India 138–143
Indian philosophy 10, 141–142, 179
Isherwood, Christopher 30, 33
Iyengar, B.K.S. 9, 10, 26, 37, 40, 41,
    43, 44, 54, 73, 82

Jainism 159, 161
Jalandhara Bandha 126
Janson, Cathie 11
Jnana Mudra 127
Jnana Yoga 37, 182
Jung, Carl Gustav 15, 134, 186

Kandinsky, Vasily 166
Kapalabhati 129
Karma Yoga 37, 47, 183
Katha Upanishad 149
Kechari Mudra 127
knee problems 57
Krishnamacharya 14, 24, 26, 40,
    44, 48
Krishnamurti 32, 33
Kriya Yoga 37, 182–183
Kriyas 126
Kumbaka 129
Kumbh Mela festival 17, 18
Kundalini serpent 27
Kundalini Yoga 37, 48, 180
Kurmasana 108–109

Laya Yoga 37
Leadbeater, Charles 31, 32
lengthening 68
limbs of yoga 65, 131
Locust 57, 96
Lord of the Dance 102–103
Lotus 92, 114–115, 128
Lotus Backbend in Shoulderstand 90–91
Lotus in Headstand 11
Lotus Twist 116–117
Lunge 118

Mahabharata 151, 153–154
Maharishi Mahesh Yogi 20, 42–44, 54
Main, John 132, 134
Mandukya Upanishad 149
Mantra Yoga 37
Mantras 132, 134
martial arts 59, 67
Mascaro, Juan 153
May, Simon 33–34
Meditation 130–135
Menuhin, Yehudi 43
Monkey 60
Mountain 57, 74–75, 78, 92, 95, 118
Mudras 127
Mula Bandha 127

Natarajasana 102–103
Nield-Smith, Penny 10
nirvana 160, 161
Niyama 172, 175

obstacles to happiness 170
Olcott, Henry 30
OM 134
Ouspensky 32

Padmasana 114–117
Paschimottanasana 100, 106–107
Patanjali 30, 48, 65, 70, 123, 131,
    161, 162, 164, 166, 170–172,
    174, 179
paths of Yoga 37
Pattabhi Jois 26, 37, 44, 48, 49
Pigeon 100–101
Pilates 60–61
Pindasana 110–111
Plough 56
power yoga 24, 37
prakrti 164, 166
prana 21, 123
Pranayama 65, 122–129, 172, 176
Pratyahara 172, 176
purusha 164

Qi Gong 59, 60

Raja Yoga 37, 154, 172, 182
Rajasic foods 54
Ram Mohan 186

Ramayana 151, 156–157
Redfield, James 34
Rg Veda 145, 148, 162
ritual chanting 15

safe practice guidelines 70–71, 73
Salabhasana 96
Salamba Sarvangasana 88–89, 90, 92
Salute to the Sun 47, 56, 111,
    118–119
Samadhi 131, 134, 172, 176
Sanmukhi mudra 56
Sanskrit terms, glossary 188
Sattvic foods 54–55
Savasana 57, 71, 120–121
Scaravelli, Vanda 26, 44–45, 47, 70,
    82–83
schools of Yoga 37
Self and ego, difference 171
Shankara 149
shoulder and neck tension 57
Shoulderstand 52, 56, 57, 88–89, 90,
    92, 116, 127
Shri Yantra 165
Siddha meditation 33
Siddha Yoga 40, 162
Sikhism 39, 139
Sirsasana 92–93
Sitting Forward bend 57
Sitting Twist 104–105
Sivananda Yoga 37, 46–47
Smakhya System 164
Spalding, Laird T. 34
spine 68–69
Spine corkscrew 52
Steiner, Rudolf 30, 31, 32
Stewart, Mary 9, 11, 26, 45, 47, 124
stress 57
stretching 86
Supta Kurmasana 108
Surya Namaskar 118–119

T'ai Chi 15, 24, 58, 59, 60, 67
Tadasana 74–75, 78, 92, 95, 118
Tamsaic foods 54
Tantric Yoga 37, 180–181
Taoist exercise system 70
Tattrirya Upanishad 148
"the One" 162, 166–169

Theosophical Society 29–32, 229, 166
therapeutic yoga 51–52
3HO 48
Thunderbolt 57
Tortoise 108–109
Transcendental Meditation (TM)
    20, 43–44
Tree 9, 56, 76–77
Triangle 56, 57, 78–79, 81
Trichur Pooram festival 143
Trikonasna 78–79, 81

Uddiyana Bandha 126
Ujayii 129
Upanishads 148–149, 153, 154, 186
Upavista Konasana 57
Urdhva Dhanurasana 82–83, 98–99
Urdhva Kukkutasana 95
Urdhva Padmasana In Sarvangasna
    90–91

varicose veins 57
Vedanta 162
Vedas 144–149, 154, 161
Viniyoga 44
Virabhadrasana 53
Vogue 7
Vrksasana 76–77

Warrior 53, 56, 81
Weil, Andrew 124
Wing Chun 59

Yama 172, 175
Yantras 134
yoga classes 10, 15, 17
yoga merchandise 17, 26
yoga schools 36–49
Yoga Sutras 30, 70, 162
Yogatattva 37
Yogi Bhajan 48

Zen art 164

THE SPIRIT OF YOGA

First edition for the United States, its dependencies, and the Philippine Islands published 2002 by Barron's Educational Series, Inc.

First published in Great Britain in 2001 by Cassell & Co.

All inquiries should be addressed to:
Barron's Educational Series, Inc.
250 Wireless Boulevard
Hauppauge, New York 11788
http://www.barronseduc.com

Library of Congress Catalog Card No.:
2001056661

International Standard Book No.:
0-7641-5512-1

Printed and bound in Italy
9 8 7 6 5 4 3 2 1

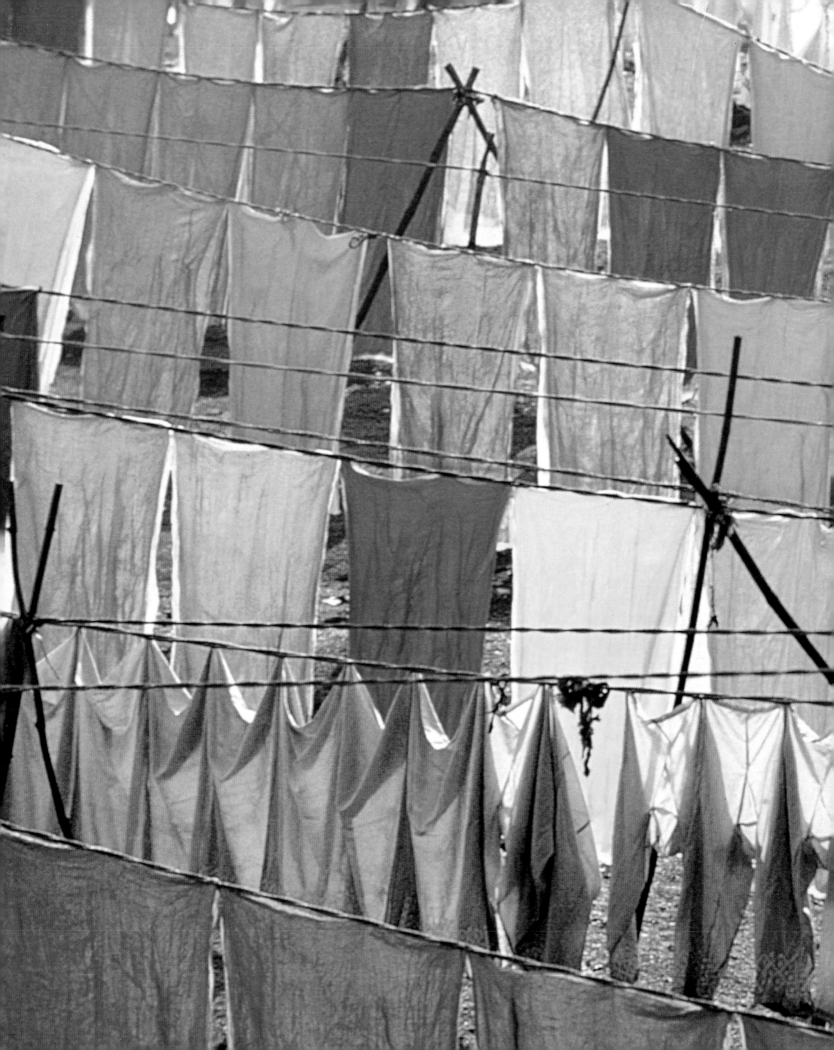